DEFYING DUCHENNE: CONQUERING CHALLENGES AND EMBRACING HOPE

DUCHENE MUSCULAR DYSTROPHY

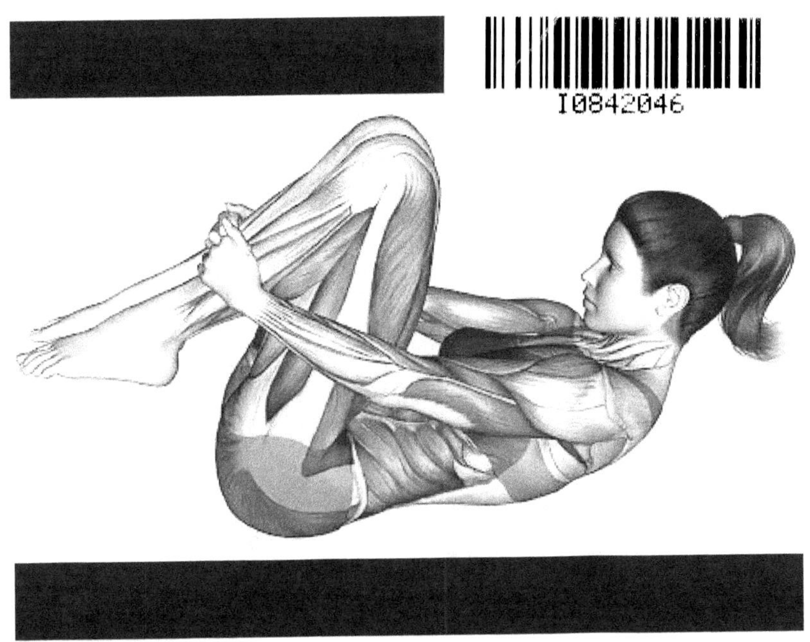

Muhammad Edogi

The views expressed in this book are solely those of the author and do not necessarily reflect the views of the publisher or any affiliated individuals or organizations.

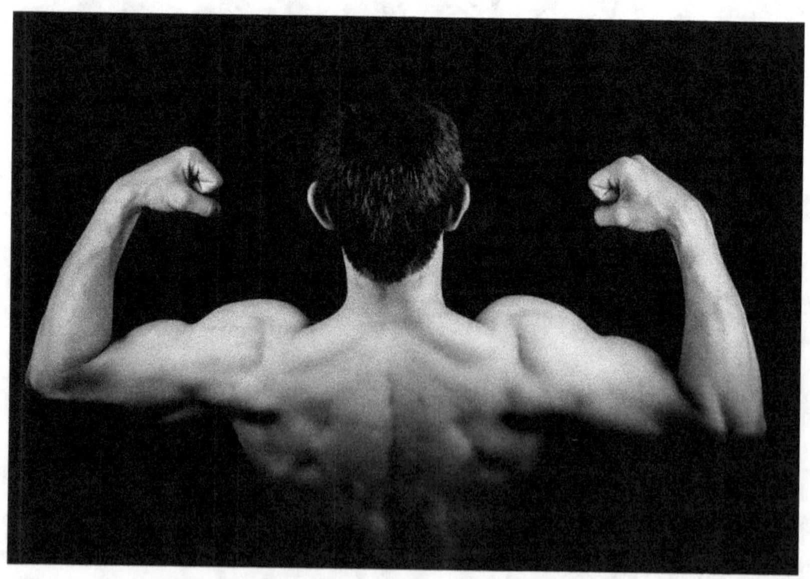

Table of Contents

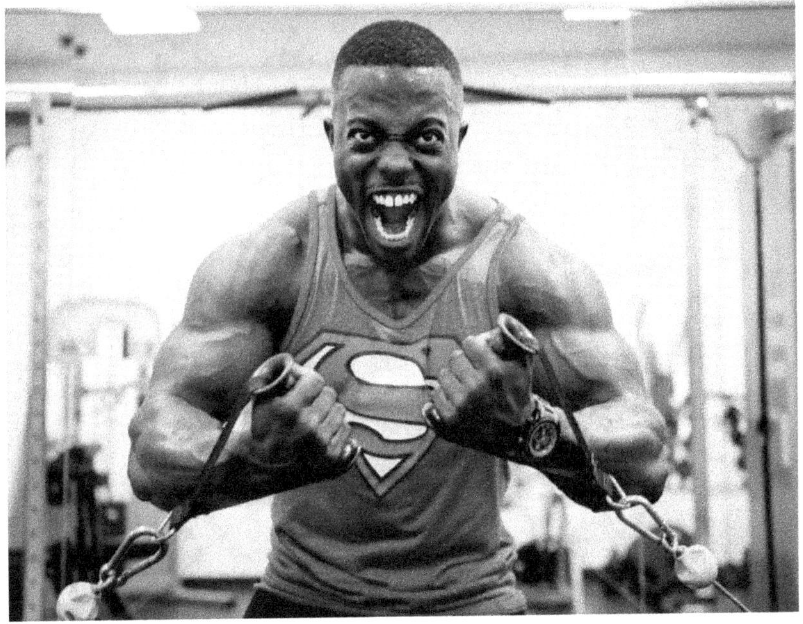

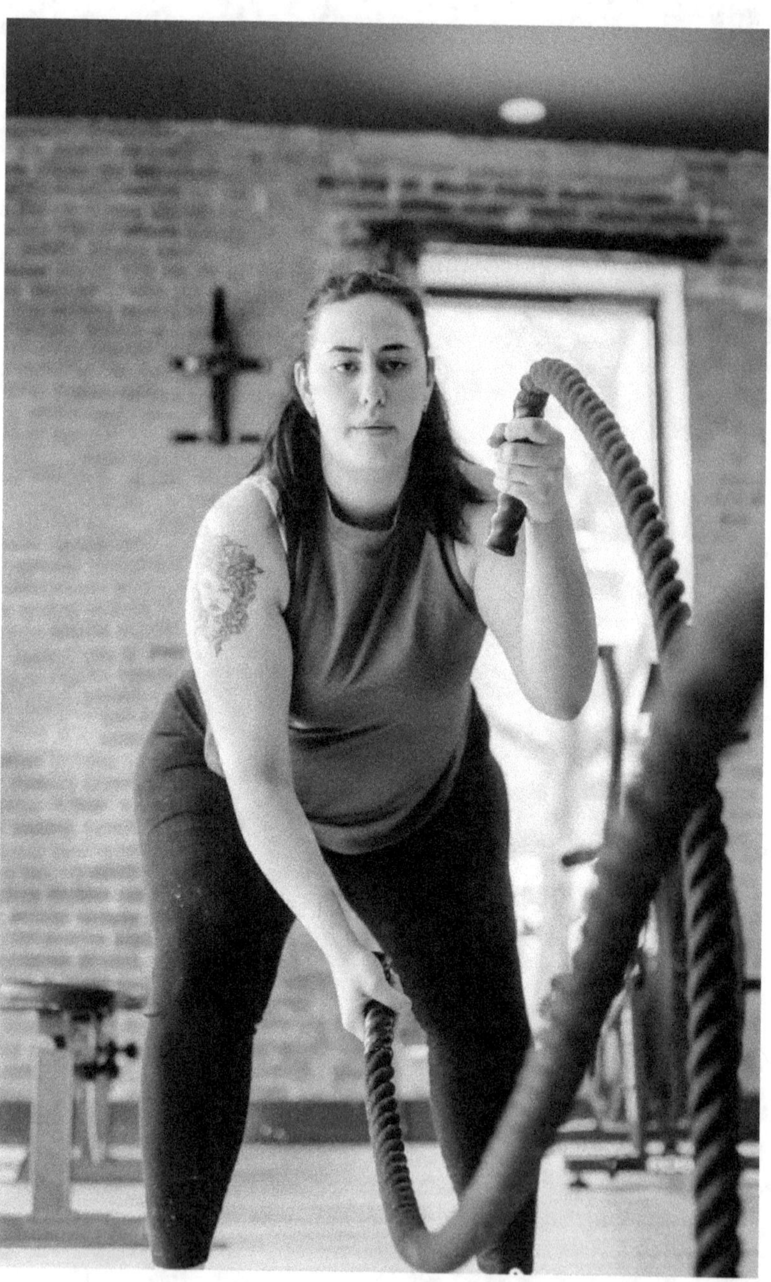

Introduction

Duchenne muscular dystrophy (DMD) is a genetic disorder that primarily affects males, causing progressive muscle weakness and degeneration. It is one of the most common and severe forms of muscular dystrophy, occurring in approximately 1 in every 3,500 to 5,000 male births worldwide.

DMD is caused by a mutation in the gene that encodes for the protein dystrophin. Dystrophin plays a crucial role in maintaining the structural integrity of muscle fibers. In individuals with DMD, the absence or deficiency of dystrophin leads to the progressive breakdown and loss of muscle tissue.

Signs and symptoms of Duchenne muscular dystrophy typically become evident in early childhood, usually between the ages of 3 and 5. Children with DMD may initially exhibit delayed motor milestones, such as late walking or difficulty in getting up from the floor. As the disease progresses, muscle weakness becomes more apparent, affecting the legs, pelvis, arms, and eventually the respiratory muscles.

The progressive nature of DMD results in increasing muscle weakness and functional impairment over time. Children may experience difficulties in walking, running, climbing stairs, and performing activities that require muscle strength. Muscle contractures, where tendons and muscles become tight and restrict joint movement, are also common in DMD.

In addition to skeletal muscle involvement, DMD can affect the heart and respiratory muscles. Cardiomyopathy, a weakening of the heart muscle, develops in most individuals with DMD by their teenage years and can lead to heart failure. Respiratory complications arise as the disease progresses, often requiring assistance with breathing using ventilatory support.

Duchenne muscular dystrophy is an X-linked recessive disorder, meaning the faulty gene is located on the X chromosome. Since males have one X chromosome and females have two, the condition predominantly affects males. However, in rare cases, females can also be carriers or exhibit milder symptoms due to skewed X-chromosome inactivation.

There is currently no cure for Duchenne muscular dystrophy, and the disease ultimately leads to significant disability and reduced life expectancy. However, advancements in research and medical interventions have improved the management of symptoms, prolonging lifespan and enhancing the quality of life for individuals with DMD.

Multidisciplinary care, including physical therapy, respiratory support, medications, orthopedic interventions, and cardiac management, aims to address the various aspects of the disease and optimize functional abilities. Ongoing research focuses on developing innovative therapies, such as gene editing and exon skipping, to target the underlying genetic defect and potentially provide more effective treatments in the future.

Overall, Duchenne muscular dystrophy is a complex and challenging condition that impacts the lives of individuals and their families. Increased awareness, early diagnosis, and comprehensive care are essential for managing the symptoms, promoting mobility, and enhancing the well-being of those affected by DMD.

Meet Alex, a five-year-old boy who has recently been diagnosed with Duchenne muscular dystrophy (DMD). Alex's parents noticed that he was having difficulty keeping up with his peers during playtime and had trouble climbing stairs. Concerned about his delayed walking and frequent falls, they sought medical advice and received the diagnosis.

Duchenne muscular dystrophy is a genetic disorder caused by a mutation in the gene that produces the dystrophin protein. In Alex's case, this mutation leads to the absence or deficiency of dystrophin in his muscle fibers. Without dystrophin, his muscles gradually weaken and degenerate over time.

As Alex grows older, his muscle weakness will progress, affecting his ability to perform everyday activities. Walking, running, and even getting up from the floor will become increasingly challenging. Alex may also develop muscle contractures, causing tightness in his joints and limiting his range of motion.

Duchenne muscular dystrophy not only affects skeletal muscles but also has implications for the heart and respiratory system. As he enters his teenage years, Alex may develop cardiomyopathy, weakening his heart muscle and potentially leading to heart failure. Additionally, the progressive weakness of his respiratory muscles may require respiratory support, such as using a ventilator, to assist with breathing.

Although Duchenne muscular dystrophy currently has no cure, Alex's healthcare team takes a multidisciplinary approach to manage his condition. Physical therapy is essential to maintain his muscle function and mobility, while medications may help slow down disease progression. Regular cardiac assessments and interventions aim to monitor and manage potential heart complications. Alex's respiratory function is closely monitored, and if necessary, he may receive respiratory support to ensure proper breathing.

While living with Duchenne muscular dystrophy poses significant challenges, ongoing research offers hope for innovative treatments. Scientists are exploring gene therapies, such as exon skipping and gene editing, which have shown promise in addressing the genetic defect underlying DMD. These emerging therapies could potentially provide more effective treatments and improve outcomes for individuals like Alex in the future.

For now, Alex's parents and caregivers focus on providing him with the best possible care and support. They connect with support organizations, learn about coping strategies, and seek educational accommodations to help him thrive academically. They also emphasize the importance of creating a positive and inclusive environment for Alex, where he can feel empowered and supported in navigating his journey with Duchenne muscular dystrophy.

Definition and Overview of Duchenne Muscular Dystrophy (DMD):

Duchenne muscular dystrophy (DMD) is a genetic disorder characterized by progressive muscle weakness and degeneration. It is named after the French neurologist Guillaume Duchenne, who first described the condition in the mid-19th century. DMD primarily affects males, although in rare cases, females can also be affected.

The key feature of DMD is the absence or deficiency of a protein called dystrophin, which is crucial for maintaining the structural integrity of muscle fibers. Dystrophin is produced by the DMD gene located on the X chromosome. Mutations in this gene result in the production of either a nonfunctional or insufficient amount of dystrophin.

Due to its X-linked recessive inheritance pattern, DMD predominantly affects males. Females have two X chromosomes, providing a protective effect if one of the X chromosomes carries the DMD mutation. However, females can be carriers of the mutated gene and have a 50% chance of passing it on to their children.

DMD typically becomes apparent in early childhood, between the ages of 3 and 5. The initial signs often include delayed motor milestones, such as late walking or difficulty in getting up from the floor. As the disease progresses, muscle weakness becomes more pronounced and affects various muscle groups, including the legs, pelvis, and upper body.

Children with DMD may exhibit a waddling gait, walk on their toes, or have difficulty climbing stairs. As they grow older, muscle weakness extends to the arms, making tasks like lifting objects or raising the arms challenging. Muscle contractures may develop, causing tightness and limiting joint mobility.

In addition to skeletal muscle involvement, DMD can impact other systems in the body. Cardiomyopathy, characterized by the weakening of the heart muscle, is a common complication and can lead to heart failure. Respiratory muscles may also weaken over time, resulting in respiratory difficulties and the potential need for respiratory support.

Duchenne muscular dystrophy is a progressive condition with no known cure. However, advancements in medical care and interventions have improved the management of symptoms and extended the lifespan of individuals with DMD. Multidisciplinary care, including physical therapy, respiratory support, orthopedic interventions, and cardiac management, aims to optimize quality of life and functional abilities.

Ongoing research focuses on developing innovative treatments, such as gene therapies and exon skipping, to address the underlying genetic defect and potentially provide more effective therapeutic options. While the challenges of living with DMD are significant, advancements in research and comprehensive care offer hope for improved outcomes and better quality of life for individuals affected by this condition.

Duchenne muscular dystrophy has a rich historical background that spans several centuries. Here are key milestones and notable figures in the understanding and recognition of this genetic disorder:

The condition now known as Duchenne muscular dystrophy was first described by the French neurologist Guillaume-Benjamin-Amand Duchenne in the 1860s. He conducted extensive clinical and pathological investigations, particularly focusing on muscle disorders.

Duchenne recognized a distinct and severe form of muscular dystrophy that predominantly affected boys and proposed the name "progressive muscular atrophy" for this condition.

Duchenne's groundbreaking work involved using electromyography (EMG) to study muscle function, and he identified specific muscle abnormalities in affected individuals.

In the 1980s, significant advancements were made in understanding the genetic basis of Duchenne muscular dystrophy.

Louis M. Kunkel, a geneticist, and his team discovered a specific gene called DMD on the X chromosome that was responsible for Duchenne and Becker muscular dystrophy.

Through their research, Kunkel's team identified the protein encoded by the DMD gene, which they named dystrophin. They found that the absence or deficiency of dystrophin led to the development of DMD.

Differentiation from Becker Muscular Dystrophy:
In the early years, Duchenne and Becker muscular dystrophies were often considered as a single entity due to their similarities. However, over time, distinctions between the two disorders emerged.

It was recognized that Becker muscular dystrophy, which has a milder course, is caused by mutations in the same DMD gene but with residual production of partially functional dystrophin protein.

The differentiation between Duchenne and Becker muscular dystrophy became clearer, helping to guide diagnoses and understanding of the two related conditions.

The latter half of the 20th century and early 21st century witnessed significant strides in the diagnosis, management, and research of Duchenne muscular dystrophy.

Improved techniques for genetic testing and identification of specific mutations in the DMD gene have enhanced the accuracy and efficiency of diagnosing DMD.

The understanding of the complex genetics and molecular mechanisms underlying DMD has led to the development of potential therapeutic approaches, such as gene therapies, exon skipping, and other innovative interventions.

While the historical background of Duchenne muscular dystrophy encompasses critical milestones, it is important to acknowledge the ongoing efforts of researchers, clinicians, and organizations dedicated to improving the lives of individuals affected by this condition. Through continued research and advancements in medical care, there is hope for further progress in the understanding and management of Duchenne muscular dystrophy.

Causes and Genetics of Duchenne Muscular Dystrophy (DMD):

Duchenne muscular dystrophy is primarily caused by mutations in the DMD gene, which is located on the X chromosome. Here are the key points regarding the causes and genetics of DMD:

1. Genetic Mutation:

Duchenne muscular dystrophy is an X-linked recessive disorder, meaning it is inherited in a recessive manner and primarily affects males.

The DMD gene provides instructions for producing the dystrophin protein, which is essential for maintaining the structural integrity of muscle fibers.

Mutations in the DMD gene disrupt the production of functional dystrophin or result in its absence, leading to muscle degeneration and weakness characteristic of DMD.

2. Dystrophin Protein:

Dystrophin is a large protein that plays a critical role in stabilizing muscle cells and protecting them from damage during muscle contraction and relaxation.

It connects the internal cytoskeleton of muscle fibers to the surrounding extracellular matrix, maintaining the integrity of the muscle cell membrane.

Types of Mutations:

Various types of mutations can occur in the DMD gene, leading to DMD. The most common mutation is the deletion of one or more exons (segments of DNA) within the gene.

Other types of mutations include duplications, insertions, or point mutations (single nucleotide changes).

The location and nature of the mutation influence the severity and clinical presentation of the disease.

> ➢ **Inheritance Pattern:**

Males have one X chromosome and one Y chromosome, while females have two X chromosomes.

Since DMD is an X-linked disorder, males who inherit a mutated copy of the DMD gene from their carrier mother will develop the disease.

Females typically have two copies of the DMD gene, and if one copy is mutated, they are carriers of DMD. In rare cases, females can exhibit symptoms if both copies of the DMD gene are mutated or if there is skewed X-chromosome inactivation.

Carrier females have a 50% chance of passing the mutated DMD gene to their children.

➤ Genetic Testing:

Genetic testing, including DNA analysis and sequencing of the DMD gene, can identify mutations responsible for DMD.

Prenatal testing, such as chorionic villus sampling or amniocentesis, can be performed to detect DMD mutations during pregnancy.

➤ Genetic Counseling:

Genetic counseling is crucial for individuals and families affected by DMD to understand the inheritance pattern, implications, and potential risks associated with the condition.

Genetic counselors provide information, support, and guidance to help individuals make informed decisions regarding family planning and genetic testing.

Understanding the causes and genetics of Duchenne muscular dystrophy is fundamental for accurate diagnosis, genetic counseling, and ongoing research efforts aimed at developing targeted therapies and interventions to address the underlying genetic defect.

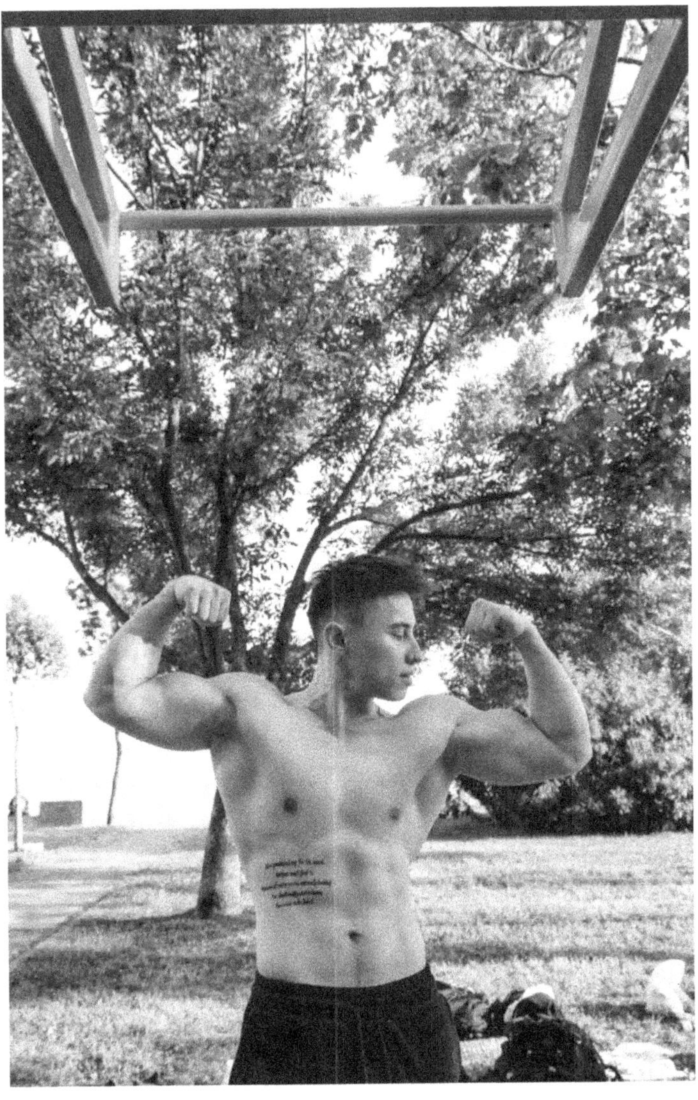

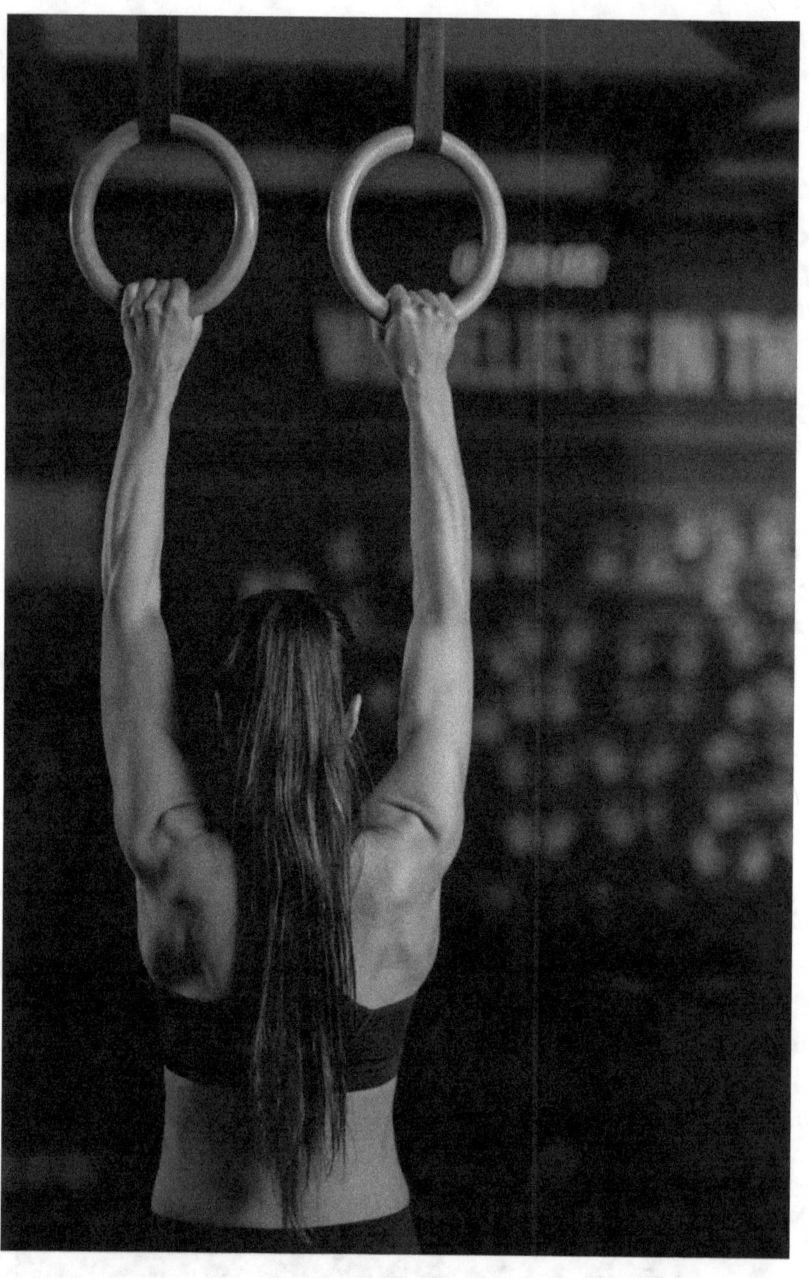

Prevalence and Inheritance Patterns of Duchenne Muscular Dystrophy (DMD):

Prevalence:

Duchenne muscular dystrophy (DMD) is one of the most common and severe forms of muscular dystrophy.

- ✓ The prevalence of DMD is estimated to be approximately 1 in every 3,500 to 5,000 male births worldwide.
- ✓ The disorder affects all ethnic groups and geographic regions, without significant variation based on race or nationality.
- ✓ Inheritance Pattern:
- ✓ Duchenne muscular dystrophy follows an X-linked recessive inheritance pattern.
- ✓ The DMD gene responsible for the disorder is located on the X chromosome.
- ✓ Females have two X chromosomes, while males have one X and one Y chromosome.
- ✓ In males, the presence of a single copy of the mutated DMD gene on the X chromosome is sufficient to cause the disease.
- ✓ Females with one mutated DMD gene are carriers and typically do not exhibit symptoms due to the presence of a second normal copy of the gene.

- ✓ Carrier females have a 50% chance of passing the mutated DMD gene to their children in each pregnancy.
- ✓ Sons of carrier females have a 50% chance of inheriting the mutated gene and developing DMD.
- ✓ Daughters of carrier females have a 50% chance of inheriting the mutated gene and becoming carriers themselves.

Expression in Carrier Females:

While carrier females typically do not develop symptoms of DMD, they can exhibit mild manifestations or have an increased risk of certain muscle-related issues.

Some carrier females may experience muscle weakness, elevated creatine kinase levels, or cardiac abnormalities.

In rare cases, carrier females can exhibit more severe symptoms if they have skewed X-chromosome inactivation, which results in a higher proportion of cells expressing the mutated gene.

➢ **New Mutations:**

In a small percentage of cases, DMD can occur due to new mutations in the DMD gene, rather than being inherited from a carrier mother.

These cases arise from spontaneous genetic changes during the formation of egg or sperm cells or during early embryonic development.

It is important to note that while DMD predominantly affects males, females play a critical role as carriers in passing on the mutated gene. Genetic counseling and testing are valuable tools for understanding the inheritance pattern, assessing the risk of having an affected child, and providing support and guidance to individuals and families affected by Duchenne muscular dystrophy.

Muscles are crucial components of the human body, enabling movement, providing support, and facilitating various physiological functions. To understand Duchenne muscular dystrophy (DMD), it is important to have a basic understanding of the structure and function of muscles.

➢ **Structure of Muscles:**

Muscles are composed of specialized cells called muscle fibers. These fibers are elongated and multinucleated, meaning they contain multiple nuclei within a single cell. Each muscle fiber is encased by a thin layer of connective tissue called the endomysium.

Muscle fibers are organized into bundles called fascicles, which are surrounded by a thicker connective tissue layer known as the perimysium. Fascicles are further grouped together, along with blood vessels and nerves, within a larger connective tissue sheath called the epimysium. This organization allows muscles to contract as a coordinated unit.

Muscles are further divided into two main types: skeletal muscles and smooth muscles. Skeletal muscles are responsible for voluntary movements, such as walking and lifting objects, and are the primary muscles affected in DMD. Smooth muscles, found in organs such as the digestive tract and blood vessels, are responsible for involuntary movements.

> **Function of Muscles:**

Muscles play a vital role in enabling movement and generating force. When a muscle contracts, its fibers shorten, resulting in the generation of force that can be transmitted to the bones and other structures. This force allows for the movement of body parts, such as bending the arm or lifting a leg.

Muscles are connected to bones via tendons, which are strong fibrous tissues that transmit the force generated by muscle contractions. When a muscle contracts, it pulls on the tendon, causing the attached bone to move.

In addition to movement, muscles are involved in various other functions, including maintaining posture, stabilizing joints, regulating body temperature, and supporting vital bodily processes such as respiration and circulation.

> **Muscle Contraction:**

Muscle contraction is a complex process involving the interaction between proteins within the muscle fibers. The basic unit of muscle contraction is the sarcomere, which is a repeating structural unit found along the length of muscle fibers.

Sarcomeres contain two types of protein filaments: thick filaments made of myosin and thin filaments composed of actin. During muscle contraction, these filaments slide past each other, resulting in the shortening of the sarcomere and overall muscle fiber.

This sliding filament model of muscle contraction is regulated by calcium ions released from specialized storage sites within the muscle fibers. The presence of calcium allows for the interaction between myosin and actin, enabling muscle contraction to occur.

Understanding the structure and function of muscles provides a foundation for comprehending the impact of Duchenne muscular dystrophy on muscle physiology. With this background, we can explore the role of dystrophin protein and how mutations in the dystrophin gene lead to DMD.

Signs and Symptoms of Duchenne Muscular Dystrophy (DMD):

Duchenne muscular dystrophy (DMD) is characterized by a progressive and predictable pattern of muscle weakness and degeneration. The signs and symptoms of DMD typically become evident in early childhood. Let's explore the early clinical manifestations of DMD:

➤ Delayed Motor Milestones:

One of the initial signs of DMD is a delay in achieving motor milestones. Children with DMD may start walking later than expected, usually between 15 and 18 months of age. Some may exhibit difficulties in standing up from a sitting or lying position. These delays are often noticeable to parents and caregivers and can be the first indication of a potential problem.

➤ Gait Abnormalities:

As DMD progresses, children may develop distinctive gait abnormalities. They may exhibit a waddling gait characterized by an exaggerated sway of the hips while walking. Another common gait abnormality observed in DMD is walking on the toes (toe-walking), which can contribute to an unsteady and imbalanced gait pattern.

> **Frequent Falls:**

Children with DMD often experience increased episodes of falling. This is due to progressive muscle weakness, particularly in the lower limbs, leading to decreased stability and coordination. The weakening of the muscles involved in balance and posture can make it challenging for children with DMD to maintain an upright position and navigate their surroundings confidently.

> **Muscle Weakness:**

Muscle weakness is a hallmark symptom of DMD and tends to progress over time. Initially, it predominantly affects the proximal muscles (closer to the center of the body), such as those in the hips and thighs. As the disease advances, the weakness extends to other muscle groups, including the upper limbs and trunk. Muscle weakness can impact a child's ability to perform various tasks, such as lifting objects, climbing stairs, or rising from the floor.

> **Enlarged Calves:**

A physical characteristic often observed in children with DMD is the enlargement of the calf muscles.

This enlargement, known as pseudohypertrophy, is due to the replacement of muscle tissue with fat and connective tissue. Although the calf muscles appear larger, they are functionally weak and demonstrate progressive muscle degeneration.

➢ **Gower's Sign:**

Gower's sign is a classic clinical finding in DMD. When attempting to rise from a seated or supine position, children with DMD often rely on their hands and arms to "walk up" their own body, using their hands to push against their thighs, abdomen, and knees. This compensatory movement is indicative of the weakness in the lower limb muscles.

It is important to note that these early clinical manifestations of DMD can vary in severity and onset from one individual to another. While some children may present with noticeable signs at a young age, others may have more subtle symptoms that become apparent as they grow older. It is crucial for parents, caregivers, and healthcare professionals to be vigilant and seek medical evaluation if they observe any of these signs or have concerns about a child's motor development. Early detection and intervention can contribute to improved management and outcomes for individuals with Duchenne muscular dystrophy.

Duchenne muscular dystrophy (DMD) is a progressive condition, meaning that the symptoms worsen and new manifestations develop over time. Understanding the progression of symptoms in DMD is important for managing the condition and providing appropriate care. Let's explore how the symptoms of DMD progress over time:

➢ **Early Childhood (Ages 3-5):**

During early childhood, the initial signs of DMD, such as delayed motor milestones and gait abnormalities, become more pronounced. Children may experience difficulties with activities that require muscle strength, such as running, jumping, and climbing. Muscle weakness primarily affects the proximal muscles, including those in the hips and thighs. Children may exhibit a waddling gait, toe-walking, and have a tendency to fall frequently.

➢ **Middle Childhood (Ages 6-12):**

As children with DMD enter middle childhood, muscle weakness progresses and starts to affect a broader range of muscles. They may struggle with tasks that involve upper limb movements, such as lifting objects, pushing, and pulling. The weakness extends to the muscles in the trunk, making it challenging to maintain an upright posture and balance. Muscle contractures, characterized by the tightening of muscles and tendons, may begin to develop, leading to joint stiffness and limited range of motion.

> **Adolescence (Ages 13-18):**

During adolescence, the symptoms of DMD typically become more severe. Muscle weakness continues to progress, impacting both the upper and lower limbs. Mobility becomes increasingly challenging, and children may require assistive devices, such as wheelchairs or mobility scooters, to move around. The weakness of respiratory muscles becomes more apparent, and respiratory complications may arise, potentially necessitating respiratory support, such as non-invasive ventilation (NIV) or mechanical ventilation.

> **Cardiac Complications:**

DMD is associated with cardiomyopathy, which refers to the weakening of the heart muscle. Cardiac involvement typically becomes evident during late childhood or adolescence. Cardiomyopathy in DMD progresses over time, potentially leading to heart failure. Monitoring cardiac function through regular assessments, such as echocardiograms and electrocardiograms, is crucial for managing cardiac complications and implementing appropriate interventions.

> **Respiratory Challenges:**

The progressive weakness of respiratory muscles significantly impacts respiratory function in individuals with DMD. Breathing difficulties become more pronounced, and respiratory support may be required to ensure adequate ventilation. This can involve non-invasive methods, such as the use of bilevel positive airway pressure (BiPAP), or, in more advanced stages, mechanical ventilation through a tracheostomy. Regular assessments of respiratory function and pulmonary care are essential to maintain optimal respiratory health.

Overall, the progression of symptoms in DMD leads to increasing functional limitations and a decline in the ability to perform daily activities independently. However, it's important to note that the rate of disease progression can vary among individuals. Regular medical monitoring, multidisciplinary care, and appropriate interventions, including physical therapy, orthopedic interventions, and respiratory support, aim to manage the symptoms, maximize quality of life, and support individuals with DMD throughout their journey.

Cardiac Involvement and Complications in Duchenne Muscular Dystrophy (DMD):

Duchenne muscular dystrophy (DMD) is not solely a disorder of skeletal muscles but also affects the heart muscle, leading to various cardiac complications. Understanding the cardiac involvement in DMD is crucial for timely diagnosis, proactive management, and optimal care. Let's explore the cardiac aspects of DMD:

➢ **Cardiomyopathy:**

One of the primary cardiac manifestations in DMD is the development of cardiomyopathy. Cardiomyopathy refers to the weakening and degeneration of the heart muscle, impairing its ability to pump blood effectively. In DMD, cardiomyopathy typically occurs during late childhood or adolescence.

➢ **Progressive Cardiac Dysfunction:**

Cardiomyopathy in DMD progresses over time, resulting in the gradual decline of cardiac function. The cardiac muscle becomes progressively weaker and less able to pump blood efficiently throughout the body. This can lead to symptoms such as fatigue, shortness of breath, and exercise intolerance.

> **Dilated Cardiomyopathy:**

The most common form of cardiomyopathy observed in DMD is dilated cardiomyopathy (DCM). In DCM, the chambers of the heart become enlarged and the walls of the heart muscle become thinner. This leads to reduced contractility and compromised pumping ability of the heart.

> **Left Ventricular Dysfunction:**

In DMD, the left ventricle, which is responsible for pumping oxygenated blood to the body, is predominantly affected. The left ventricular dysfunction contributes to the reduced cardiac output and can lead to symptoms such as breathlessness, fluid retention, and eventually heart failure.

> **Arrhythmias:**

Arrhythmias, irregular heart rhythms, can occur in individuals with DMD. These abnormal heart rhythms can be caused by the structural and electrical changes within the heart muscle. Arrhythmias can manifest as palpitations, dizziness, fainting, or even sudden cardiac arrest. Regular cardiac monitoring, including electrocardiograms (ECGs), helps detect and manage arrhythmias.

> **Risk of Sudden Cardiac Death:**

Individuals with DMD have an increased risk of sudden cardiac death. The weakening of the heart muscle and the presence of arrhythmias contribute to this risk. Implementing appropriate cardiac surveillance, including regular cardiac assessments and monitoring, is essential to identify potential risks and intervene as necessary.

> **Cardiac Management:**

Optimal cardiac management in DMD involves a multidisciplinary approach and regular monitoring. This may include:

Cardiac assessments: Regular echocardiograms, ECGs, and cardiac MRI scans to evaluate cardiac structure and function.

Medications: Certain medications, such as angiotensin-converting enzyme (ACE) inhibitors or beta-blockers, may be prescribed to manage cardiac function and delay the progression of cardiomyopathy.

Cardiac devices: In some cases, implantable devices like pacemakers or implantable cardioverter-defibrillators (ICDs) may be recommended to manage arrhythmias and provide appropriate treatment in emergency situations.

Cardiac rehabilitation: Tailored exercise programs and physical activity guidance to maintain cardiac health and optimize functional capacity.

Overall, cardiac involvement and complications are significant aspects of DMD. Regular cardiac evaluations, proactive management, and close collaboration between the medical team and individuals with DMD and their families are crucial in monitoring and addressing cardiac issues, thereby enhancing the overall care and quality of life for individuals affected by DMD.

Respiratory Implications and Challenges in Duchenne Muscular Dystrophy (DMD):

Duchenne muscular dystrophy (DMD) is not limited to skeletal muscle weakness but also affects the muscles involved in respiration. Respiratory complications are a significant aspect of DMD, and understanding the respiratory implications is crucial for managing the condition effectively. Let's explore the respiratory challenges faced by individuals with DMD:

> **Progressive Respiratory Muscle Weakness:**

Progressive muscle weakness in DMD affects the muscles responsible for breathing, including the diaphragm and intercostal muscles. As these muscles weaken, respiratory function becomes compromised, leading to various challenges.

> **Reduced Vital Capacity:**

Vital capacity refers to the maximum amount of air a person can exhale after taking a deep breath. In DMD, vital capacity decreases as respiratory muscles weaken. This reduction in vital capacity affects the ability to take in an adequate volume of air, leading to decreased oxygen levels and impaired lung function.

➢ **Respiratory Insufficiency:**

As DMD progresses, respiratory insufficiency can develop, characterized by an inability to maintain sufficient oxygenation and elimination of carbon dioxide. This insufficiency can lead to symptoms such as shortness of breath, fatigue, and decreased exercise tolerance.

➢ **Difficulty with Coughing and Clearing Secretions:**

Weakened respiratory muscles make it challenging for individuals with DMD to generate a forceful cough and effectively clear respiratory secretions. Inefficient coughing and ineffective secretion clearance can result in the accumulation of mucus and potential respiratory infections, such as pneumonia.

➢ **Sleep-Disordered Breathing:**

Sleep-disordered breathing is common in DMD. It includes various conditions such as nocturnal hypoventilation, obstructive sleep apnea, and central sleep apnea. Respiratory muscle weakness can contribute to abnormal breathing patterns during sleep, leading to fragmented sleep, excessive daytime sleepiness, and impaired overall respiratory function.

> **Respiratory Support and Interventions:**

Respiratory support and interventions are essential for managing respiratory challenges in DMD. The following approaches may be implemented:

Non-Invasive Ventilation (NIV):

Non-invasive ventilation, such as the use of bilevel positive airway pressure (BiPAP) or non-invasive positive pressure ventilation (NIPPV), assists with breathing by providing mechanical support during sleep or periods of respiratory distress. NIV can help maintain sufficient oxygenation and improve overall respiratory function.

> **Mechanical Ventilation:**

In advanced stages of DMD, as respiratory function further declines, individuals may require full-time mechanical ventilation. This involves the use of a ventilator and a tracheostomy tube to assist with breathing. Mechanical ventilation helps ensure adequate oxygenation and ventilation to support life.

> **Assisted Cough Techniques:**

To aid in secretion clearance, assisted cough techniques can be employed. These techniques, such as manually assisted coughing or mechanical insufflation-exsufflation devices, help generate an effective cough and clear respiratory secretions.

> ### Regular Pulmonary Assessments:

Regular assessments of pulmonary function, such as spirometry, peak cough flow, and arterial blood gas analysis, are crucial for monitoring respiratory function, identifying changes, and guiding interventions.

> ### Pulmonary Rehabilitation:

Pulmonary rehabilitation programs, which include exercise, breathing exercises, and education, can help optimize respiratory function, improve exercise tolerance, and enhance overall quality of life.

Respiratory challenges are progressive in DMD, and close monitoring, proactive management, and timely interventions are crucial. Regular respiratory assessments, respiratory support devices, and pulmonary rehabilitation play vital roles in maintaining optimal respiratory health and enhancing the well-being of individuals with DMD.

Diagnosis and Genetic Testing for Duchenne Muscular Dystrophy

4.1 Medical History and Physical Examination

Duchenne Muscular Dystrophy (DMD) is a severe, progressive neuromuscular disorder that primarily affects boys. The diagnosis of DMD involves a comprehensive medical history and physical examination, which are essential for identifying clinical features and assessing disease progression. Additionally, genetic testing plays a crucial role in confirming the diagnosis and determining the specific genetic mutation responsible for the condition.

4.1.1 Medical History

Obtaining a detailed medical history is the initial step in the diagnostic process for DMD. The healthcare provider will interview the patient and their family members to gather information about the individual's developmental milestones, motor function, and any concerning symptoms or family history of neuromuscular disorders. Key aspects of the medical history may include:

> **Milestone Development:** The physician will inquire about the age at which the child achieved motor milestones such as crawling,

walking, and running. Delayed achievement or regression of these milestones may be indicative of a neuromuscular disorder like DMD.

- ➢ **Gait Abnormalities:** Parents or caregivers may be asked to describe any abnormalities observed in the child's gait, such as frequent falls, difficulty getting up from the floor, or a characteristic "waddling" gait pattern.

- ➢ **Muscle Weakness:** Inquiring about muscle weakness in various muscle groups, including the limbs, trunk, and neck, is crucial. Providers will often ask about difficulties with activities such as climbing stairs, lifting objects, or raising the arms overhead.

- ➢ **Respiratory Function:** Evaluating respiratory symptoms is essential, as respiratory muscle weakness is a common feature of DMD. Providers will ask about signs of breathing difficulties, such as shortness of breath, rapid breathing, or frequent respiratory infections.

- ➢ **Cardiac Involvement:** DMD is also associated with cardiac abnormalities. Questions about symptoms such as chest pain, palpitations, or unexplained fatigue may be asked to assess potential cardiac involvement.

- ➢ **Family History:** Obtaining a comprehensive family history is vital, as DMD is an X-linked disorder. Inquiring about affected relatives, consanguinity, or any other neuromuscular disorders in the family helps identify potential genetic risk factors.

4.1.2 Physical Examination

After gathering the medical history, a thorough physical examination is conducted to assess the presence and extent of muscle weakness and other clinical signs of DMD. The examination typically involves:

> **Musculoskeletal Examination:** The physician will assess muscle bulk, strength, and tone in different muscle groups. They may perform manual muscle testing to evaluate the strength of specific muscles. In DMD, proximal muscles are usually more affected than distal muscles. The child may exhibit signs such as Gowers' sign, which involves using the hands to push against the legs while rising from a squatting position.

> **Gait Analysis:** Observing the child's gait pattern is important. Children with DMD often exhibit a waddling gait due to weakness in the pelvic and hip muscles. They may have difficulty walking on their heels and exhibit an exaggerated lordotic posture.

- **Contractures:** Contractures, characterized by the shortening of muscles and tendons, are common in DMD. The physician will examine for joint contractures, particularly in the ankles, knees, and elbows, which can restrict mobility.
- **Neurological Examination:** The provider will assess other neurological functions such as deep tendon reflexes, sensory perception, and coordination. While intellectual development is typically unaffected in DMD, cognitive assessments may also be performed to rule out associated conditions.
- **Cardiac Evaluation:** Due to the risk of cardiac involvement, a thorough cardiac examination may be conducted, including auscultation for murmurs, palpation for the presence of a cardiac impulse, and assessing heart sounds.
- **Respiratory Assessment:** Evaluation of respiratory function is critical. The physician may listen for abnormal breath sounds, assess respiratory rate, and measure oxygen saturation. In advanced stages of DMD, respiratory muscle weakness may lead to respiratory insufficiency.

4.1.3 Role of Medical History and Physical Examination in Diagnosis

The medical history and physical examination serve as essential tools for the diagnosis of DMD. Clinical features such as delayed or regressed motor milestones, muscle weakness, abnormal gait, contractures, and respiratory or cardiac symptoms raise suspicion of the disorder. These findings, combined with a comprehensive family history, provide valuable clues for the diagnosis of DMD.

While the medical history and physical examination are informative, they do not provide a definitive diagnosis. Genetic testing is required to confirm the presence of DMD and identify the specific genetic mutation responsible for the disorder. Therefore, genetic testing is an integral part of the diagnostic process for DMD and will be discussed in the subsequent section.

In addition to medical history, physical examination, and genetic testing, laboratory tests and biomarkers play a significant role in the diagnosis and monitoring of Duchenne Muscular Dystrophy (DMD). These tests provide valuable information about muscle function, disease progression, and potential complications associated with DMD.

➤ 4.2.1 Creatine Kinase (CK) Levels

Elevated serum creatine kinase (CK) levels are a hallmark laboratory finding in individuals with DMD. CK is an enzyme found predominantly in skeletal muscle, and its release into the bloodstream is indicative of muscle damage or breakdown. In DMD, the absence or deficiency of the dystrophin protein leads to muscle fiber degeneration and subsequent release of CK into circulation. Therefore, measuring CK levels can be a useful screening tool for suspected cases of DMD.

Typically, CK levels in individuals with DMD are significantly elevated, often exceeding ten times the upper limit of the normal range. However, it is important to note that elevated CK levels can also be observed in other conditions involving muscle damage, such as inflammatory myopathies or other muscular dystrophies. Therefore, further diagnostic tests, such as genetic testing, are necessary to confirm the diagnosis of DMD.

> ## 4.2.2 Muscle Biopsy

Muscle biopsy involves the removal of a small sample of muscle tissue for microscopic examination. Although it is an invasive procedure, muscle biopsy can provide important diagnostic information in cases where genetic testing is inconclusive or not available.

In DMD, muscle biopsy reveals characteristic pathological features, including the presence of muscle fiber degeneration, infiltration of fat and connective tissue, and the absence or reduction of dystrophin protein expression. Immunohistochemistry staining can be performed to visualize dystrophin protein levels and assess its distribution within muscle fibers.

While muscle biopsy can aid in diagnosing DMD, it is generally reserved for cases where genetic testing does not provide a definitive diagnosis or when additional information is needed for research purposes or therapeutic interventions.

> ## 4.2.3 Electrodiagnostic Studies

Electro diagnostic studies, such as electromyography (EMG) and nerve conduction studies (NCS), can be helpful in assessing muscle and nerve function in individuals with DMD.

EMG measures the electrical activity of muscles at rest and during voluntary muscle contractions. In DMD, EMG findings may reveal myopathic changes, characterized by short, small-amplitude, and polyphasic motor unit potentials. These changes reflect muscle fiber degeneration and can help differentiate between muscle and nerve involvement.

NCS assesses the integrity and function of peripheral nerves. In DMD, NCS is typically normal unless there is concurrent peripheral neuropathy or involvement of nerve roots. Therefore, NCS is not routinely performed in the diagnosis of DMD but may be used to evaluate coexisting nerve pathology or differential diagnosis.

> ### 4.2.4 Biomarkers

Biomarkers are measurable substances or indicators that can provide information about a particular biological process or disease state. In DMD, various biomarkers have been investigated to monitor disease progression, assess therapeutic efficacy, and predict potential complications.

One of the most studied biomarkers in DMD is serum levels of the N-terminal fragment of the prohormone brain natriuretic peptide (NT-proBNP). NT-proBNP is primarily released by the ventricular myocardium in response to cardiac stress. Elevated NT-proBNP levels have been associated with the onset and progression of cardiomyopathy in DMD. Regular monitoring of NT-proBNP levels can help detect early cardiac involvement and guide appropriate cardiac management strategies.

Another biomarker of interest is serum levels of myostatin, a protein that negatively regulates muscle growth. Increased myostatin levels have been observed in individuals with DMD, contributing to muscle wasting and weakness. Monitoring myostatin levels may provide insights into disease progression and the effectiveness of potential therapeutic interventions targeting myostatin.

Furthermore, emerging biomarkers, such as muscle-specific microRNAs (miRNAs), are being investigated in DMD. miRNAs are small non-coding RNA molecules that regulate gene expression. Specific miRNA signatures have shown promise in predicting disease progression, identifying therapeutic targets, and monitoring treatment response in DMD.

4.2.5 Other Laboratory Tests

Additional laboratory tests may be performed to evaluate organ function and monitor potential complications associated with DMD. These tests may include:

> **Cardiac evaluations:** Electrocardiogram (ECG) and echocardiography to assess cardiac structure and function.

> **Pulmonary function tests:** Spirometry and respiratory muscle strength measurements to assess respiratory function.

> **Serum electrolyte levels:** Monitoring for imbalances or abnormalities, such as potassium or calcium levels.

> **Liver function tests:** Evaluating liver enzymes to assess liver health and potential liver involvement.

> **Renal function tests:** Measuring serum creatinine and assessing kidney function.

These laboratory tests, in conjunction with clinical assessments and imaging studies, contribute to a comprehensive evaluation of individuals with DMD and help monitor disease progression, detect potential complications, and guide appropriate management strategies.

In laboratory tests and biomarkers, including serum CK levels, muscle biopsy, electrodiagnostic studies, and various biomarkers, play an important role in the diagnosis and management of Duchenne Muscular Dystrophy. These tests provide valuable information about muscle function, disease progression, and potential complications associated with DMD, aiding in accurate diagnosis, monitoring of disease course, and guiding appropriate treatment and supportive care strategies.

Genetic testing plays a crucial role in the diagnosis of Duchenne Muscular Dystrophy (DMD) by identifying specific genetic mutations responsible for the disorder. There are several genetic testing methods available, each with its own advantages and limitations. The following are some of the commonly used genetic testing methods for DMD:

Polymerase Chain Reaction (PCR): PCR is a widely used technique in genetic testing for DMD. It allows for the amplification of specific regions of the dystrophin gene, making it easier to identify mutations. PCR can be used to detect small point mutations or sequence variations in the gene.

Multiplex Ligation-dependent Probe Amplification (MLPA): MLPA is a technique used to detect deletions or duplications of one or more exons in the dystrophin gene. It involves hybridizing specific probes to the DNA, followed by amplification and analysis. MLPA can detect large-scale deletions or duplications, which are common in DMD.

Sanger Sequencing: Sanger sequencing is a traditional method used for DNA sequencing. It allows for the determination of the exact nucleotide sequence of the dystrophin gene. Sanger sequencing is useful for identifying small mutations or sequence variations, including single-nucleotide substitutions or small insertions/deletions.

Next-Generation Sequencing (NGS): NGS technologies have revolutionized genetic testing by enabling the rapid and cost-effective sequencing of large portions of the genome. NGS can be used for targeted gene panel sequencing or whole exome sequencing (WES). Targeted gene panel sequencing focuses on specific genes of interest, including the dystrophin gene, and provides a more focused analysis. WES involves sequencing all the protein-coding regions of the genome and can provide a broader analysis of genetic variants.

Array Comparative Genomic Hybridization (aCGH): aCGH is a technique used to detect copy number variations, such as deletions or duplications, in the dystrophin gene. It involves comparing the patient's DNA to a reference DNA sample and analyzing the hybridization pattern. aCGH can identify large-scale deletions or duplications in the gene.

Whole Genome Sequencing (WGS): WGS is a comprehensive genetic testing method that sequences the entire genome. It provides a detailed analysis of an individual's genetic information, including the dystrophin gene. WGS can identify various types of genetic mutations, including point mutations, insertions, deletions, and structural variants. However, WGS is a more costly and time-consuming approach compared to targeted sequencing methods.

It is important to note that the choice of genetic testing method depends on several factors, including the availability of resources, the suspected mutation type, and the clinical presentation. In some cases, multiple testing methods may be used in combination to achieve a definitive diagnosis.

In addition to these specific genetic testing methods, it is also worth mentioning that other techniques, such as fluorescent in situ hybridization (FISH), array-based comparative genomic hybridization (aCGH), and multiplex PCR, may be utilized for research or specific diagnostic purposes.

In genetic testing methods for Duchenne Muscular Dystrophy (DMD) include PCR, MLPA, Sanger sequencing, next-generation sequencing (NGS), array comparative genomic hybridization (aCGH), and whole genome sequencing (WGS). These methods allow for the identification of genetic mutations in the dystrophin gene, aiding in the diagnosis and genetic characterization of individuals with DMD. The choice of testing method depends on factors such as the suspected mutation type and available resources.

Prenatal diagnosis and genetic counseling play a crucial role in the management and support of families affected by Duchenne Muscular Dystrophy (DMD). These processes provide valuable information about the genetic status of the fetus, facilitate informed decision-making, and offer support to individuals and families throughout the diagnostic and reproductive planning stages.

4.4.1 Prenatal Diagnosis

Prenatal diagnosis involves the identification of DMD in a fetus during pregnancy. It allows parents to obtain early and accurate information about the genetic status of the unborn child, enabling them to make informed decisions regarding pregnancy management, treatment options, and future family planning.

There are several prenatal diagnostic methods available for DMD:

Chorionic Villus Sampling (CVS): CVS is typically performed between the 10th and 12th weeks of pregnancy. It involves the removal of a small sample of chorionic villi, which are cells from the placenta that contain the same genetic information as the fetus. The sample is then analyzed using genetic testing methods, such as PCR or DNA sequencing, to detect the presence of DMD mutations.

Amniocentesis: Amniocentesis is usually performed between the 15th and 20th weeks of pregnancy. During this procedure, a small amount of amniotic fluid, which contains fetal cells, is extracted from the amniotic sac surrounding the fetus. The fetal cells are then analyzed using genetic testing methods to determine the presence of DMD mutations.

Prenatal genetic testing methods, such as PCR, DNA sequencing, or deletion/duplication analysis, are used to identify specific mutations in the dystrophin gene in the fetus. The results of these tests provide valuable information about the genetic status of the fetus, allowing parents to plan for appropriate medical care and support after birth.

It is important to note that prenatal diagnosis carries a small risk of pregnancy loss due to the invasive nature of the procedures. Genetic counseling should be offered to parents to help them understand the benefits, risks, and limitations of prenatal testing and make informed decisions.

4.4.2 Genetic Counseling

Genetic counseling is an integral part of the diagnostic and management process for DMD. It provides individuals and families with information, support, and guidance regarding the genetic aspects of the condition. Genetic counseling sessions are typically conducted by healthcare professionals trained in genetics and counseling.

Genetic counseling for DMD involves the following components:

- ❖ **Discussion of Family History:** The genetic counselor will gather detailed information about the family history, including any known cases of DMD or other neuromuscular disorders. This information helps assess the risk of DMD and provides insight into potential genetic carriers within the family.
- ❖ **Explanation of DMD Genetics:** The genetic counselor will explain the inheritance pattern of DMD, which is an X-linked recessive disorder. They will discuss how the dystrophin gene is passed down from parents to children, the risk of having an affected child, and the chances of passing on the condition to future generations.
- ❖ **Explanation of Diagnostic Testing:** The genetic counselor will explain the different

genetic testing methods available for DMD diagnosis, including their benefits, limitations, and possible outcomes. They will discuss the option of prenatal diagnosis for families planning future pregnancies and provide information about the procedures involved and the associated risks.

- ❖ **Interpretation of Genetic Test Results**: If genetic testing has been performed, the genetic counselor will interpret the results and explain the implications for the individual or family. They will discuss the specific genetic mutation identified, the associated symptoms and prognosis, and potential treatment and management options.
- ❖ **Psychosocial Support and Resources:** Genetic counseling provides emotional support to individuals and families coping with the diagnosis of DMD. The counselor can help address concerns, provide coping strategies, and connect families with support groups and resources specific to DMD.
- ❖ **Reproductive Options and Family Planning:** Genetic counseling assists families in making informed decisions about family planning and reproductive options. The counselor will discuss the various options available, such as prenatal diagnosis, preimplantation genetic

diagnosis (PGD), adoption, or the use of assisted reproductive technologies.

Genetic counseling sessions are tailored to the specific needs of each family and may involve multiple sessions to address various aspects of the condition and its impact on the family's life. The goal of genetic counseling is to empower individuals and families with knowledge and support, enabling them to make informed decisions and navigate the challenges associated with DMD.

Prenatal diagnosis and genetic counseling are essential components of the management and support provided to individuals and families affected by Duchenne Muscular Dystrophy. Prenatal diagnosis allows for early detection of DMD in the fetus, enabling parents to make informed decisions about pregnancy management and future family planning. Genetic counseling provides individuals and families with information, support, and guidance regarding the genetic aspects of DMD, including diagnostic testing, inheritance patterns, treatment options, and psychosocial support. Together, prenatal diagnosis and genetic counseling contribute to improved care, decision-making, and overall well-being for families affected by DMD.

Management and Treatment Approaches

5.1 Multidisciplinary Care and Team Approach

Effective management of Duchenne Muscular Dystrophy (DMD) requires a comprehensive and coordinated approach involving a multidisciplinary care team. The complex nature of DMD necessitates the involvement of various healthcare professionals with specialized expertise in different aspects of the disorder. This team-based approach ensures optimal care, addresses the diverse needs of individuals with DMD, and promotes the best possible outcomes. The following healthcare professionals may be involved in the multidisciplinary care of individuals with DMD:

Pediatrician/Primary Care Physician: The pediatrician or primary care physician serves as the central point of contact and coordinates overall care. They monitor general health, provide routine vaccinations, manage common illnesses, and coordinate referrals to specialists.

Neurologist: A neurologist with expertise in neuromuscular disorders, such as DMD, plays a critical role in the diagnosis, assessment, and ongoing management of the disease. They evaluate motor function, monitor disease progression, prescribe medications, and provide guidance on supportive care strategies.

Genetic Counselor: Genetic counselors provide information, support, and counseling to individuals and families regarding the genetic aspects of DMD. They explain the inheritance pattern, discuss genetic testing options, and provide guidance for family planning.

Physiotherapist: Physiotherapy plays a central role in the management of DMD. Physiotherapists develop and implement personalized exercise programs to maintain muscle strength, flexibility, and range of motion. They also provide respiratory physiotherapy to optimize lung function, prescribe mobility aids, and assist with adaptive equipment.

Occupational Therapist: Occupational therapists help individuals with DMD maintain independence and improve their ability to perform daily activities. They provide guidance on adaptive strategies, recommend assistive devices, and assess and address any difficulties in fine motor skills and activities of daily living.

Cardiologist: Cardiac involvement is a significant concern in DMD. Cardiologists monitor cardiac function, perform regular assessments (including electrocardiograms and echocardiograms), prescribe medication to manage cardiac complications, and provide guidance on cardiac surveillance and management.

Pulmonologist: Respiratory muscle weakness is a progressive feature of DMD. Pulmonologists assess respiratory function, monitor lung health, prescribe respiratory interventions (such as cough assistance devices, non-invasive ventilation, or invasive ventilation if required), and provide guidance on respiratory management and infection prevention.

Orthopedic Surgeon: Orthopedic surgeons manage orthopedic complications that may arise due to muscle weakness, such as contractures and scoliosis. They may perform surgical procedures, including tendon releases, spinal fusion, or corrective surgeries, to optimize mobility and maintain the best possible musculoskeletal function.

Nutritionist/Dietitian: Nutritionists or dietitians provide guidance on optimal nutrition and dietary management in DMD. They address any issues related to growth, weight management, bone health, and gastrointestinal symptoms, ensuring individuals receive adequate nutrition to support muscle function and overall well-being.

Speech and Language Therapist: Speech and language therapists assist individuals with DMD who may experience difficulties with speech, swallowing, and communication. They provide strategies to enhance communication skills, recommend adaptations to diet and feeding techniques, and address any speech or swallowing difficulties.

Psychologist/Social Worker: Psychologists or social workers provide psychosocial support to individuals with DMD and their families. They help address emotional well-being, coping strategies, adjustment to diagnosis, and facilitate access to support groups and community resources.

Education Specialist: Education specialists collaborate with schools and educators to support the educational needs of individuals with DMD. They develop individualized education plans (IEPs), recommend accommodations or assistive technology, and ensure a supportive learning environment.

The multidisciplinary care team works collaboratively, sharing information, expertise, and treatment plans to optimize the overall management of DMD. Regular team meetings and communication facilitate coordinated care and ensure that all aspects of the individual's health and well-being are addressed.

Additionally, the care team collaborates with individuals and families to develop personalized care plans, set treatment goals, and provide education and resources for managing the disease effectively at home. Regular follow-up visits and ongoing communication between team members and families are essential to monitor disease progression, address concerns, and adjust management strategies as needed.

A multidisciplinary care approach involving various healthcare professionals is crucial for the effective management of Duchenne Muscular Dystrophy. This team-based approach ensures comprehensive care, addresses the diverse needs of individuals with DMD, and optimizes outcomes by providing specialized expertise and coordinated management across multiple domains of health and well-being.

The management of Duchenne Muscular Dystrophy (DMD) includes the use of medications and drug therapies aimed at slowing disease progression, managing symptoms, and improving quality of life. While there is no cure for DMD, several medications have shown beneficial effects in delaying disease progression and addressing specific aspects of the disorder. The following are some of the commonly used medications and drug therapies in the management of DMD:

Corticosteroids (Glucocorticoids): Corticosteroids, such as prednisone and deflazacort, are the mainstay of pharmacological treatment for DMD. These medications have been shown to slow the progression of muscle weakness and preserve muscle function. Corticosteroids work by reducing inflammation, decreasing muscle damage, and increasing muscle strength. They are typically started in the early stages of the disease and continued throughout the lifespan. However, long-term use of corticosteroids is associated with side effects, including weight gain, growth retardation, osteoporosis, and behavioral changes. The dose and duration of corticosteroid therapy should be carefully monitored and individualized.

Exon Skipping Therapies: Exon skipping is an emerging therapeutic approach that aims to restore the reading frame of the dystrophin gene. This approach utilizes medications such as eteplirsen, golodirsen, and viltolarsen, which are administered via intravenous infusion. These drugs target specific genetic mutations in DMD and help promote the production of a partially functional dystrophin protein. Exon skipping therapies have shown improvements in motor function and the preservation of muscle strength in some individuals with specific genetic mutations. Regular monitoring for treatment efficacy and potential side effects is necessary.

Nonsense Mutation Readthrough Therapy: Nonsense mutation readthrough therapy involves the use of medications, such as ataluren, to enable the translation of dystrophin protein even in the presence of premature stop codons caused by specific genetic mutations. This therapy aims to restore a functional dystrophin protein and potentially slow disease progression. Ataluren is administered orally and has shown modest benefits in a subset of individuals with specific genetic mutations. Regular monitoring and close collaboration with a healthcare provider are essential for treatment optimization.

Cardiac Medications: Given the high risk of cardiac complications in DMD, specific medications may be prescribed to manage cardiac function and delay the onset of cardiomyopathy. Angiotensin-converting enzyme (ACE) inhibitors, such as enalapril and lisinopril, or angiotensin receptor blockers (ARBs), such as losartan, are commonly prescribed to help reduce cardiac strain and slow the progression of heart dysfunction. Beta-blockers, such as carvedilol or metoprolol, may also be used to manage heart rate and blood pressure. Regular cardiac evaluations and monitoring are crucial to adjust medication dosages and ensure optimal management of cardiac function.

Respiratory Medications: As respiratory muscle weakness is a progressive aspect of DMD, respiratory medications are often prescribed to manage respiratory function and prevent complications. Medications such as bronchodilators (e.g., albuterol), inhaled corticosteroids, and mucolytics (e.g., acetylcysteine) may be used to manage airway inflammation, bronchospasm, and excessive mucus production. Non-invasive ventilation (NIV) devices, such as bilevel positive airway pressure (BiPAP) or continuous positive airway pressure (CPAP), may be prescribed to support breathing during sleep and reduce the risk of respiratory failure.

Pain Management: Individuals with DMD may experience pain, particularly related to muscle and joint complications. Nonsteroidal anti-inflammatory drugs (NSAIDs), such as ibuprofen, may be prescribed to manage pain and reduce inflammation. Physical therapy, occupational therapy, and other non-pharmacological pain management strategies may also be employed to address pain symptoms.

It is important to note that the use of medications and drug therapies in DMD should be individualized based on the specific needs and characteristics of each person. The risks and benefits of treatment options, including potential side effects, should be carefully considered and discussed with a healthcare provider. Regular monitoring and assessment of treatment efficacy, as well as ongoing communication with the healthcare team, are essential for optimizing medication management in DMD.

medications and drug therapies play a significant role in the management of Duchenne Muscular Dystrophy. Corticosteroids, exon skipping therapies, nonsense mutation readthrough therapy, cardiac medications, respiratory medications, and pain management strategies are among the commonly used pharmacological approaches. The choice of medications and treatment plans should be individualized, taking into consideration the specific needs, genetic mutations, disease progression, and potential side effects of each person with DMD. Regular monitoring, close collaboration with healthcare providers, and ongoing evaluation of treatment efficacy are essential for optimizing medication management in DMD.

Physical therapy and rehabilitation play a critical role in the management of Duchenne Muscular Dystrophy (DMD). These interventions aim to optimize physical function, maintain mobility, prevent complications, and enhance overall quality of life. A comprehensive physical therapy and rehabilitation program is tailored to the specific needs of individuals with DMD, taking into account their age, disease progression, functional abilities, and individual goals. The following are key aspects of physical therapy and rehabilitation in DMD:

Exercise and Strengthening Programs: Physical therapists develop individualized exercise programs to maintain muscle strength, flexibility, and range of motion. These programs often involve a combination of stretching, strengthening exercises, and low-impact aerobic activities. Exercises focus on preserving functional abilities, improving posture, and preventing contractures. They may include resistance training, manual stretching, and activities that promote cardiovascular fitness.

Assistive Devices and Mobility Aids: Physical therapists assess and prescribe appropriate assistive devices and mobility aids to maximize mobility and independence. These may include orthotics (such as ankle-foot orthoses), braces, canes, walkers, wheelchairs, or powered mobility devices. Assistive devices help compensate for muscle weakness, improve stability, and enhance overall functional abilities.

Gait Training and Mobility Skills: Gait training aims to optimize walking abilities and improve overall mobility. Physical therapists work with individuals to optimize their gait pattern, develop compensatory strategies, and use assistive devices effectively. They may also provide training in activities such as transfers, stair climbing, and safe mobility within the community.

Respiratory Management: Respiratory physiotherapy is an essential component of DMD management. Physical therapists provide strategies and exercises to optimize respiratory function, maintain chest wall mobility, and prevent respiratory complications. Techniques may include deep breathing exercises, airway clearance techniques, and assistance with non-invasive ventilation (NIV) devices.

Postural Management and Scoliosis Prevention: Individuals with DMD are at increased risk of developing scoliosis due to muscle weakness. Physical therapists assess postural alignment, provide recommendations for maintaining proper posture, and develop strategies to prevent or delay the progression of scoliosis. They may prescribe postural exercises, recommend orthotic devices, and collaborate with orthopedic surgeons if surgical intervention is required.

Pain Management and Modalities: Physical therapists may employ various modalities and techniques to manage pain associated with DMD. These may include heat or cold therapy, transcutaneous electrical nerve stimulation (TENS), massage, or other pain management modalities. Additionally, they provide education on proper positioning, body mechanics, and energy conservation techniques to reduce pain and discomfort.

Education and Caregiver Training: Physical therapists educate individuals with DMD and their caregivers about the importance of exercise, mobility, and proper body mechanics. They provide guidance on performing exercises at home, using assistive devices safely, and managing activities of daily living. Caregivers are trained in proper handling techniques, transfers, and ways to optimize the physical environment to enhance accessibility and safety.

Collaboration with the Multidisciplinary Team: Physical therapists work collaboratively with other healthcare professionals involved in the care of individuals with DMD, such as occupational therapists, respiratory therapists, orthopedic surgeons, and assistive technology specialists. They actively participate in multidisciplinary team meetings, share information, and contribute to the development of comprehensive care plans.

Regular physical therapy sessions, periodic reassessment, and ongoing communication with the physical therapy team are essential for monitoring progress, adjusting interventions, and addressing changing needs as the disease progresses.

physical therapy and rehabilitation are integral components of the management of Duchenne Muscular Dystrophy. These interventions aim to optimize physical function, maintain mobility, prevent complications, and enhance overall quality of life. Through exercise programs, assistive devices, mobility training, respiratory management, and pain management strategies, physical therapy helps individuals with DMD maintain functional abilities, improve posture, and enhance independence. Collaboration with the multidisciplinary care team ensures comprehensive and coordinated care, addressing the diverse needs of individuals with DMD.

Assistive devices and mobility aids play a crucial role in supporting individuals with Duchenne Muscular Dystrophy (DMD) in maintaining mobility, independence, and overall quality of life. As muscle weakness progresses in DMD, these devices compensate for impaired strength, improve stability, and enhance functional abilities. The selection and use of appropriate assistive devices and mobility aids are tailored to the specific needs and abilities of each individual. The following are some commonly used assistive devices and mobility aids in the management of DMD:

Orthotics and Ankle-Foot Orthoses (AFOs): Orthotics and AFOs are custom-fitted devices that provide support, stabilize the ankle and foot, and improve walking ability. AFOs help compensate for foot drop and promote a more functional gait pattern. They are typically made of lightweight materials and fit inside the shoe to provide support and alignment.

Braces and Splints: Braces and splints are used to support and stabilize joints affected by muscle weakness and contractures in DMD. They may be applied to the ankles, knees, wrists, or elbows, depending on the specific needs of the individual. Braces and splints help maintain joint alignment, prevent contractures, and improve functional abilities.

Canes and Walkers: Canes and walkers provide stability and support for individuals with DMD who have difficulty walking independently. Canes help with balance and provide additional support during ambulation. Walkers, such as front-wheeled or four-wheeled walkers, offer more stability and support for individuals with greater mobility challenges. These devices improve safety, assist with weight-bearing, and help conserve energy.

Wheelchairs: Wheelchairs are often used as the primary mobility device for individuals with advanced DMD or significant mobility limitations. Manual wheelchairs require self-propulsion, while power wheelchairs are powered by an electric motor. Wheelchairs provide independence, improve mobility, and enable participation in various activities. They can be customized with features such as adjustable seating, headrests, and specialized controls to meet individual needs.

Powered Mobility Devices: Powered mobility devices, such as scooters or powered wheelchairs, are beneficial for individuals with DMD who require greater assistance with mobility. These devices offer increased range, speed, and maneuverability, allowing individuals to travel longer distances independently. Powered mobility devices provide enhanced accessibility, promote social engagement, and improve overall quality of life.

Transfer Aids: Transfer aids are devices designed to assist with safe transfers and repositioning. Examples include transfer boards, sliding sheets, and transfer poles. These aids reduce the physical strain on individuals with DMD and caregivers during transfers between different surfaces, such as beds, chairs, or vehicles.

Bathroom and Toileting Aids: Bathroom and toileting aids are designed to promote independence and safety in personal hygiene tasks. These may include grab bars, raised toilet seats, shower chairs, commode chairs, and adaptive toileting equipment. These aids provide stability, support, and accessibility, allowing individuals with DMD to maintain their dignity and independence.

Adaptive Seating and Positioning Systems: Adaptive seating and positioning systems are used to provide postural support, improve comfort, and prevent deformities associated with muscle weakness. These systems include specialized cushions, backrests, and seating inserts that promote proper alignment and pressure distribution, reducing the risk of pressure sores and optimizing sitting posture.

It is crucial to consult with healthcare professionals, such as physical therapists, occupational therapists, and assistive technology specialists, to determine the most appropriate assistive devices and mobility aids for each individual with DMD. These professionals assess functional abilities, consider disease progression, and provide guidance on proper use, maintenance, and adjustments of assistive devices to ensure optimal benefits.

Regular evaluations, adjustments, and follow-up visits with the assistive technology team are important to address changing needs, provide ongoing support, and ensure the continued effectiveness of assistive devices and mobility aids.

assistive devices and mobility aids play a significant role in enhancing mobility, independence, and overall quality of life for individuals with Duchenne Muscular Dystrophy. Orthotics, AFOs, braces, canes, walkers, wheelchairs, powered mobility devices, transfer aids, bathroom and toileting aids, adaptive seating and positioning systems are among the commonly used devices. The selection and use of these aids are individualized based on specific needs, abilities, and disease progression. Collaboration with healthcare professionals specializing in assistive technology ensures proper fitting, appropriate selection, and ongoing support to optimize mobility and independence in individuals with DMD.

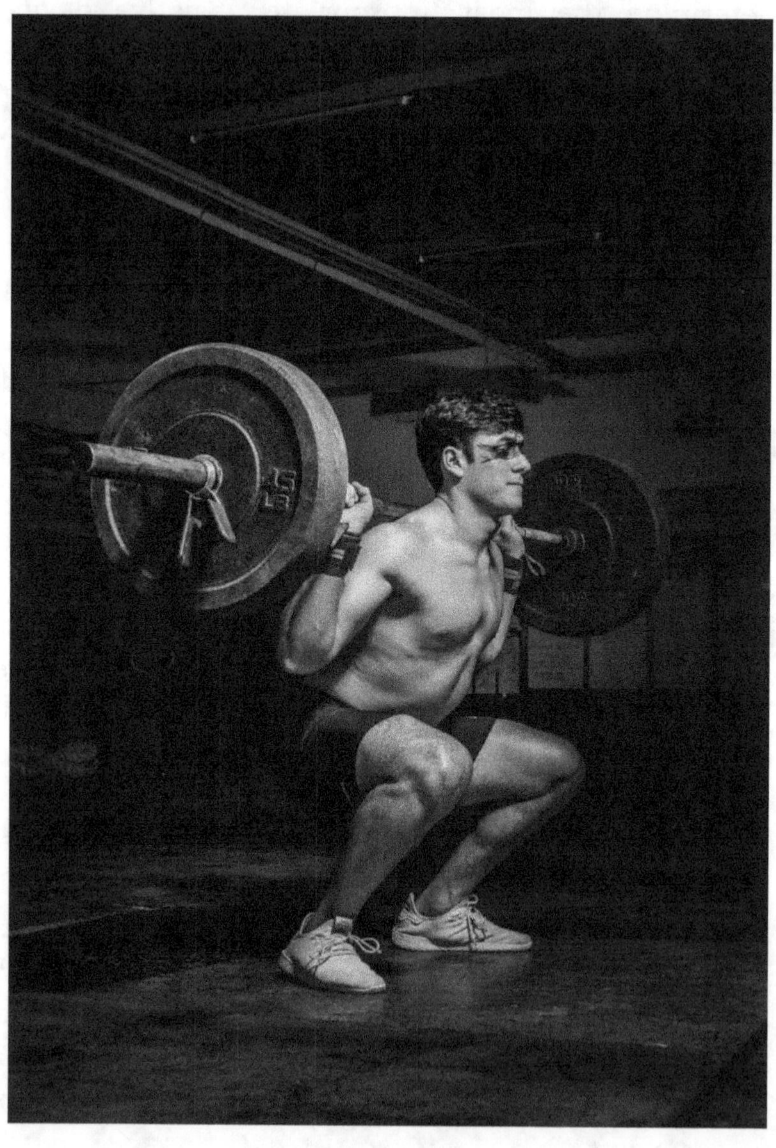

Orthopedic interventions and the management of contractures are crucial aspects of the comprehensive care for individuals with Duchenne Muscular Dystrophy (DMD). As muscle weakness progresses, individuals with DMD are at risk of developing contractures, which are permanent tightening and shortening of muscles and tendons. Contractures can significantly impact mobility, functional abilities, and overall quality of life. The following are important considerations for orthopedic interventions and the management of contractures in DMD:

Regular Monitoring and Assessment: Regular monitoring of joint range of motion, muscle strength, and flexibility is essential to detect the early signs of contractures. Healthcare professionals, such as orthopedic surgeons and physical therapists, perform assessments and measurements at regular intervals to identify the presence and severity of contractures. This allows for timely intervention and the implementation of appropriate management strategies.

Stretching and Range of Motion Exercises: Stretching exercises and range of motion exercises are crucial in the management of contractures. Physical therapists develop personalized stretching programs to maintain or improve joint flexibility and prevent the progression of contractures. These exercises target specific muscles and joints to promote lengthening, flexibility, and optimal range of motion. Stretching should be performed regularly and may be combined with other therapies, such as heat or splinting, to enhance effectiveness.

Orthotic Devices: Orthotic devices, such as braces and splints, are commonly used to manage contractures in DMD. These devices help maintain or improve joint alignment, prevent further contracture development, and promote optimal positioning. Orthotics are customized to the individual's specific needs and may be worn during certain activities or for longer durations. An orthopedic specialist or physical therapist assesses the specific joint and muscle involvement to determine the most appropriate orthotic intervention.

Serial Casting: Serial casting involves applying a series of casts to gradually stretch and lengthen contracted muscles and tendons. This method is particularly useful for individuals with more severe contractures. The cast is applied to maintain a prolonged stretch on the affected muscles and tendons, and it is periodically adjusted to progressively increase the stretching force. Serial casting is performed under the supervision of an orthopedic specialist and may be combined with other therapies, such as stretching exercises or physical therapy.

Surgical Interventions: In some cases, surgical interventions may be necessary to address severe contractures or correct skeletal deformities in individuals with DMD. Orthopedic surgeries, such as tendon releases, tendon lengthening, or corrective osteotomies, may be performed to improve joint mobility, correct alignment, and enhance functional abilities. These surgeries are typically performed by orthopedic surgeons with expertise in neuromuscular disorders and are tailored to the specific needs and goals of each individual.

Post-Operative Rehabilitation: Following orthopedic surgeries, individuals undergo post-operative rehabilitation, which includes physical therapy and rehabilitation to optimize recovery and regain functional abilities. Physical therapists develop individualized rehabilitation programs to address muscle strength, range of motion, gait training, and functional activities. The rehabilitation process is closely coordinated with the orthopedic team to ensure a comprehensive and integrated approach.

Prevention of Contractures: Preventing contractures is an essential aspect of managing DMD. Regular stretching exercises, physical therapy, and the use of orthotic devices help maintain muscle length, joint flexibility, and prevent the development of contractures. Additionally, optimizing weight management, promoting physical activity within functional limitations, and implementing strategies to manage pain and discomfort contribute to preventing contracture progression.

It is important to note that orthopedic interventions and the management of contractures should be individualized based on the specific needs, functional abilities, and disease progression of each person with DMD. Regular evaluation, monitoring, and communication with healthcare professionals specializing in orthopedics and rehabilitation are vital to develop personalized management plans, ensure the effectiveness of interventions, and address any emerging needs over time.

Orthopedic interventions and the management of contractures are integral components of comprehensive care for individuals with Duchenne Muscular Dystrophy. Regular monitoring, stretching exercises, orthotic devices, serial casting, surgical interventions, and post-operative rehabilitation contribute to maintaining joint flexibility, preventing contractures, optimizing alignment, and improving functional abilities. Collaboration with orthopedic specialists, physical therapists, and other healthcare professionals is essential to develop personalized management strategies and optimize the overall musculoskeletal health of individuals with DMD.

Cardiac and respiratory care are critical components of the management of Duchenne Muscular Dystrophy (DMD) due to the progressive involvement of the heart and respiratory muscles. Regular monitoring, early intervention, and targeted management strategies are essential in preserving cardiac and respiratory function, optimizing overall health, and improving the quality of life for individuals with DMD. The following are key considerations for cardiac and respiratory care in DMD:

> **Cardiac Care:**

a. Regular Cardiac Monitoring: Regular cardiac evaluations are essential for early detection of cardiomyopathy, the most common cardiac complication in DMD. Cardiologists monitor cardiac function through various tests, including electrocardiograms (ECGs), echocardiograms (ECHO), and cardiac MRI. Monitoring frequency and specific tests may vary based on individual needs and disease progression.

b. Medications: Cardiac medications are often prescribed to manage heart function and delay the progression of cardiomyopathy. Angiotensin-converting enzyme (ACE) inhibitors, such as enalapril or lisinopril, or angiotensin receptor blockers (ARBs), such as losartan, may be prescribed to reduce cardiac strain and promote heart health. Beta-blockers, such as carvedilol or metoprolol, can help manage heart rate and blood pressure.

c. Heart Failure Management: In advanced stages of cardiomyopathy or heart failure, additional treatments may be necessary. These may include diuretics to manage fluid retention, vasodilators to improve blood flow, or inotropic medications to enhance heart contractility. In severe cases, advanced interventions like cardiac resynchronization therapy (CRT) or heart transplantation may be considered.

d. Lifestyle Modifications: Lifestyle modifications such as maintaining a heart-healthy diet, engaging in appropriate physical activity, and avoiding tobacco and alcohol are important for overall cardiovascular health. Weight management, blood pressure control, and regular follow-ups with a cardiologist are recommended.

➢ **Respiratory Care:**

a. Pulmonary Function Monitoring: Regular monitoring of respiratory function is essential to detect changes in lung function and assess the need for interventions. Pulmonologists perform pulmonary function tests (PFTs), including spirometry, to measure lung volumes and flow rates. Peak cough flow measurements and overnight pulse oximetry may also be performed to evaluate respiratory muscle strength and nighttime oxygen saturation levels.

b. Respiratory Muscle Training: Respiratory muscle training aims to maintain or improve respiratory muscle strength. This may include exercises such as deep breathing exercises, incentive spirometry, and inspiratory muscle training. These exercises help maintain lung volumes, improve cough effectiveness, and enhance overall respiratory function.

c. Non-Invasive Ventilation (NIV): Non-invasive ventilation is often prescribed to support breathing and manage respiratory muscle weakness in DMD. Devices such as bilevel positive airway pressure (BiPAP) or continuous positive airway pressure (CPAP) provide ventilatory support during sleep or as needed. NIV helps reduce respiratory fatigue, improve gas exchange, and enhance overall respiratory function.

d. Airway Clearance Techniques: Airway clearance techniques, such as manual chest physiotherapy, positive expiratory pressure devices, or high-frequency chest wall oscillation devices, are employed to help clear excess mucus and maintain optimal airway clearance. These techniques assist in preventing respiratory infections and reducing the risk of respiratory complications.

e. Invasive Ventilation: In advanced stages of respiratory muscle weakness, invasive ventilation may be required. This may involve tracheostomy and the use of mechanical ventilators to provide continuous respiratory support. Invasive ventilation can improve quality of life, maintain adequate oxygenation, and extend survival in individuals with severe respiratory compromise.

f. Infection Prevention: Preventing respiratory infections is crucial for individuals with DMD. Vaccinations, including annual influenza vaccines and pneumococcal vaccines, are recommended. Good respiratory hygiene practices, such as frequent handwashing and avoiding exposure to sick individuals, should be followed. Prompt treatment of respiratory infections and regular follow-ups with a pulmonologist are important.

g. Palliative Care: Palliative care focuses on improving quality of life and providing supportive care for individuals with advanced DMD. Palliative care teams address pain management, symptom control, psychosocial support, and end-of-life planning. These teams collaborate with the multidisciplinary care team to ensure comprehensive care and support for individuals and their families.

Regular follow-up visits with cardiologists and pulmonologists, close monitoring of cardiac and respiratory function, and open communication with the healthcare team are essential for optimal cardiac and respiratory care in DMD. Caregivers and individuals with DMD should receive education and training regarding signs of cardiac and respiratory distress, emergency procedures, and how to appropriately use prescribed equipment and medications.

In cardiac and respiratory care are vital components of the management of Duchenne Muscular Dystrophy. Regular monitoring, medication management, lifestyle modifications, and targeted interventions such as cardiac medications, respiratory muscle training, non-invasive or invasive ventilation, and infection prevention strategies are employed to preserve cardiac and respiratory function. Collaboration with cardiologists, pulmonologists, and the multidisciplinary care team ensures comprehensive care and improved quality of life for individuals with DMD.

Psychosocial support and promoting a high quality of life are integral aspects of the comprehensive care provided to individuals with Duchenne Muscular Dystrophy (DMD) and their families. The emotional, social, and psychological well-being of individuals with DMD are equally important alongside the physical management of the condition. The following are key considerations for psychosocial support and enhancing the quality of life in DMD:

Psychosocial Counseling: Psychosocial support should be readily available to individuals with DMD and their families. Psychologists, social workers, or counselors with expertise in neuromuscular disorders provide emotional support, coping strategies, and counseling services. These professionals assist individuals and families in dealing with the emotional impact of the diagnosis, adjusting to changes, managing stress, and addressing any mental health concerns.

Support Groups: Support groups bring together individuals with DMD, their families, and caregivers facing similar challenges. These groups provide a supportive environment to share experiences, exchange information, and offer emotional support. Support groups can be in-person or online and may be organized by healthcare facilities, patient advocacy organizations, or community organizations.

Education and Information: Providing accurate and comprehensive information about DMD helps individuals and families understand the condition, its management, and available resources. Educational sessions, workshops, and access to reliable online resources enable individuals to make informed decisions, understand treatment options, and actively participate in their care.

School Support and Education: Collaboration between healthcare professionals, educators, and school administrators is essential to ensure appropriate support and accommodations for students with DMD. Individualized education plans (IEPs) and 504 plans can be developed to address academic, physical, and social needs. School-based therapists, such as occupational therapists or physical therapists, may also be involved in supporting students with DMD in the school setting.

Transition to Adulthood: The transition from pediatric to adult care can be a challenging period for individuals with DMD. Support services and resources should be available to assist in this transition, including guidance on navigating adult healthcare systems, vocational counseling, and financial planning. Collaboration between pediatric and adult healthcare providers ensures a seamless transition and continuity of care.

Assistive Technology and Accessibility: Access to appropriate assistive technology and adaptive equipment is vital for enhancing independence and quality of life. This may include communication devices, environmental control systems, accessible transportation, and home modifications. Assistive technology specialists and occupational therapists can help individuals with DMD identify and acquire the necessary devices to optimize functionality and accessibility.

Palliative and End-of-Life Care: Palliative care should be integrated into the care plan for individuals with advanced DMD. Palliative care teams address pain management, symptom control, psychosocial support, and assistance with end-of-life planning. These services ensure comfort, dignity, and support for individuals and their families throughout the disease progression.

Respite Care and Caregiver Support: Caregivers play a vital role in supporting individuals with DMD. Respite care services provide temporary relief to caregivers, allowing them to take breaks and attend to their own well-being. Caregiver support programs, such as counseling, educational resources, and support groups, help caregivers cope with the demands and challenges associated with caring for a loved one with DMD.

Encouraging Social Engagement and Inclusion: Promoting social engagement and inclusion is crucial for enhancing the quality of life of individuals with DMD. Encouraging participation in social activities, community events, and peer interactions fosters a sense of belonging and overall well-being. Adaptive sports programs and recreational activities specifically designed for individuals with disabilities can provide opportunities for socialization and physical activity.

Resilience-Building and Positive Coping Strategies: Encouraging the development of resilience and positive coping strategies helps individuals with DMD and their families navigate the challenges associated with the condition. This may involve promoting self-advocacy skills, fostering a positive mindset, encouraging open communication, and offering resources for stress management and coping techniques.

In psychosocial support and enhancing quality of life are essential components of the comprehensive care provided to individuals with Duchenne Muscular Dystrophy. Psychosocial counseling, support groups, education, school support, assistive technology, palliative care, caregiver support, social engagement, and resilience-building strategies all contribute to promoting emotional well-being, empowerment, and overall quality of life for individuals with DMD and their families. Collaborative efforts between healthcare professionals, support organizations, and the broader community are necessary to provide a holistic approach to care and support.

Emerging Therapies and Research Advances

6.1 Gene Therapies and Genetic Manipulation

In recent years, there have been significant advancements in the field of gene therapies and genetic manipulation for Duchenne Muscular Dystrophy (DMD). These emerging therapies hold great promise for the treatment of the underlying genetic cause of DMD and have the potential to transform the management and prognosis of the condition. The following are key considerations regarding gene therapies and genetic manipulation in DMD:

Gene Replacement Therapy: Gene replacement therapy aims to deliver a functional copy of the dystrophin gene to muscle cells, thereby producing a functional dystrophin protein. This approach utilizes viral vectors, such as adeno-associated viruses (AAVs), to deliver the therapeutic gene to muscle tissue. Preclinical and early clinical trials have shown promising results, with some individuals exhibiting increased dystrophin expression and improved muscle function. Ongoing research is focused on optimizing delivery methods, enhancing the duration of gene expression, and assessing long-term safety and efficacy.

Exon Skipping Therapies: Exon skipping is a genetic manipulation approach that aims to bypass specific genetic mutations in the dystrophin gene. This strategy utilizes synthetic molecules called antisense oligonucleotides (ASOs) to modulate gene expression and promote the production of shorter but partially functional dystrophin proteins. Several exon skipping therapies, such as eteplirsen, golodirsen, and viltolarsen, have been approved for specific genetic mutations in DMD. Ongoing research aims to expand the applicability of exon skipping therapies to additional genetic mutations.

Gene Editing Technologies: Gene editing technologies, such as CRISPR-Cas9, offer the potential to precisely modify the genetic sequence of the dystrophin gene. CRISPR-Cas9 allows targeted deletion, insertion, or correction of specific mutations in the DNA. While still in the early stages of development, gene editing holds promise for precise correction of genetic mutations responsible for DMD. Research efforts are focused on refining delivery methods, optimizing gene editing efficiency, and addressing potential off-target effects.

Utrophin Up regulation: Utrophin is a protein similar to dystrophin that can compensate for its absence in DMD. Utrophin up regulation strategies aim to increase the expression of utrophin in muscle cells to provide functional support. Various approaches, including small molecules and gene therapy vectors, are being explored to enhance utrophin expression and function. Preclinical studies have demonstrated the potential of utrophin up regulation as a therapeutic strategy for DMD.

Antisense Oligonucleotide-mediated Exon Inclusion: In addition to exon skipping, antisense oligonucleotides can be used to promote the inclusion of specific exons that are usually skipped in DMD. This approach aims to restore the reading frame and produce a more functional dystrophin protein. Preclinical studies have shown promising results in restoring dystrophin expression and improving muscle function. Further research is needed to optimize delivery methods and assess the safety and efficacy of exon inclusion therapies.

Combination Therapies: Researchers are exploring the potential benefits of combining different therapeutic approaches to maximize efficacy and overcome limitations. Combinations of gene therapies, exon skipping therapies, and other emerging strategies are being investigated to achieve synergistic effects and address different aspects of the disease.

It is important to note that while gene therapies and genetic manipulation hold immense potential for the treatment of DMD, these approaches are still under development and require further research and clinical trials to establish their long-term safety and effectiveness. Regulatory approvals, scalability of production, accessibility, and affordability are also important considerations in the translation of these emerging therapies to widespread clinical use.

In gene therapies and genetic manipulation represent exciting and rapidly evolving fields in the management of Duchenne Muscular Dystrophy. Advances in gene replacement therapy, exon skipping therapies, gene editing technologies, utrophin upregulation, and exon inclusion strategies offer potential avenues for treating the underlying genetic cause of DMD. Continued research and development, as well as collaboration between scientists, clinicians, regulatory bodies, and industry partners, are essential to bring these emerging therapies to fruition and improve the lives of individuals living with DMD.

Exon skipping and antisense oligonucleotide (ASO) therapy are emerging treatment approaches for Duchenne Muscular Dystrophy (DMD). These therapies aim to restore the reading frame of the dystrophin gene and promote the production of a partially functional dystrophin protein. The following are key considerations for exon skipping and ASO therapy:

Mechanism of Action: Exon skipping utilizes synthetic molecules called antisense oligonucleotides to target specific sections (exons) of the dystrophin gene. By binding to the targeted exon, the ASO promotes skipping of the exon during the RNA splicing process, allowing the production of a shorter but partially functional dystrophin protein. This approach aims to restore the reading frame and maintain muscle function.

Approved ASO Therapies: Several ASO therapies have been approved for specific genetic mutations in DMD. Eteplirsen, golodirsen, and viltolarsen target exon 51 skipping and have shown efficacy in increasing dystrophin expression and improving motor function in some individuals. These therapies are administered via intravenous infusion and require regular monitoring for treatment efficacy and potential side effects.

Expanded ASO Approaches: Research is ongoing to develop ASO therapies targeting additional exons in the dystrophin gene. ASOs targeting exons 45, 53, and 44 are currently being investigated in clinical trials. The goal is to expand the applicability of exon skipping therapies to a larger population of individuals with different genetic mutations.

Challenges and Limitations: Despite the promising results of ASO therapy, challenges remain. ASOs need to be delivered systemically to reach all affected muscle groups, which can be a challenge due to their size and ability to cross barriers. Optimization of delivery methods, such as improved systemic delivery or localized administration, is an area of active research. Additionally, the long-term effects, optimal treatment duration, and the impact on various organ systems require further investigation.

Stem cell therapy and regenerative medicine hold potential for the treatment of Duchenne Muscular Dystrophy (DMD). These approaches aim to repair or replace damaged muscle tissue and restore muscle function. The following are key considerations for stem cell therapy and regenerative medicine in DMD:

Stem Cell Sources: Different types of stem cells are being investigated for their potential in DMD treatment. Embryonic stem cells, induced pluripotent stem cells (iPSCs), and adult stem cells, such as muscle-derived stem cells and mesenchymal stem cells (MSCs), are among the cell sources being explored. Each has its advantages and limitations in terms of availability, scalability, differentiation potential, and immune compatibility.

Muscle Stem Cell Transplantation: Muscle stem cell transplantation involves the delivery of healthy muscle stem cells into affected muscles to replace damaged or dystrophic muscle fibers. These cells have the ability to regenerate and differentiate into functional muscle cells. Strategies to enhance muscle stem cell engraftment and survival are being investigated, including the use of biomaterials, growth factors, and genetic modification.

Gene-Edited Stem Cells: Gene editing technologies, such as CRISPR-Cas9, can be applied to stem cells to correct disease-causing mutations before transplantation. This approach aims to generate dystrophin-producing stem cells that can differentiate into functional muscle cells. Research is ongoing to optimize gene editing techniques, ensure safety and efficacy, and develop scalable manufacturing processes.

Exosome Therapy: Exosomes are small vesicles released by stem cells that contain various signaling molecules, growth factors, and genetic material. Exosome therapy involves the administration of exosomes derived from stem cells to promote tissue repair and regeneration. Studies have shown that stem cell-derived exosomes can enhance muscle function, reduce inflammation, and promote tissue healing in preclinical models of DMD.

Tissue Engineering and 3D Bioprinting: Tissue engineering and 3D bioprinting technologies aim to create functional muscle tissue in the laboratory for transplantation. These approaches involve combining stem cells, biomaterial scaffolds, and growth factors to generate three-dimensional muscle constructs. This field is still in its early stages, and further research is needed to refine the techniques and optimize tissue functionality.

Clinical trials play a crucial role in evaluating the safety and efficacy of new therapies for Duchenne Muscular Dystrophy (DMD). Several experimental treatments are currently being investigated, and some show promise in preclinical and early clinical studies. The following are examples of promising experimental treatments and ongoing clinical trials:

Microdystrophin Gene Therapy: Microdystrophin gene therapy aims to deliver a smaller but functional version of the dystrophin gene to muscle cells using viral vectors. Early clinical trials have shown increased dystrophin expression and improvements in muscle function in treated individuals. Further research is ongoing to optimize delivery methods, durability of gene expression, and long-term effects.

Gene Editing with CRISPR-Cas9: Gene editing technologies, such as CRISPR-Cas9, hold promise for correcting specific genetic mutations in the dystrophin gene. Preclinical studies have demonstrated successful gene editing in animal models of DMD. Clinical trials are being planned or initiated to evaluate the safety and efficacy of CRISPR-Cas9 in humans.

Utrophin Modulation: Utrophin modulation aims to increase the expression and functionality of the utrophin protein as a substitute for dystrophin. Small molecules and genetic approaches are being explored to upregulate utrophin expression and promote muscle protection and regeneration. Early preclinical and clinical studies have shown promising results, and further research is underway.

Anti-Fibrotic Therapies: Fibrosis, the excessive accumulation of connective tissue, contributes to muscle dysfunction in DMD. Anti-fibrotic therapies aim to prevent or reduce fibrosis in affected muscles. Drugs targeting fibrotic pathways, such as transforming growth factor-beta (TGF-β) inhibitors and anti-fibrotic compounds, are being investigated in preclinical and clinical trials.

Combination Therapies: Combination therapies that target multiple aspects of DMD pathology are being explored to maximize therapeutic benefits. For example, combining exon skipping therapies with anti-inflammatory drugs or muscle protectants may have synergistic effects. Clinical trials are investigating the safety and efficacy of such combination approaches.

It is important to note that while these emerging therapies and experimental treatments show promise, they are still in various stages of development and require further research and rigorous clinical testing to establish their safety and efficacy. Participation in clinical trials provides an opportunity for eligible individuals to access these innovative treatments and contribute to advancing the field.

In exon skipping and antisense oligonucleotide therapies, stem cell therapy and regenerative medicine, and promising experimental treatments offer new avenues for the treatment of Duchenne Muscular Dystrophy. Ongoing research, clinical trials, and collaborative efforts among researchers, clinicians, regulatory bodies, and patient advocacy groups are critical in advancing these therapies and improving the lives of individuals with DMD.

Living with Duchenne Muscular Dystrophy

Living with Duchenne Muscular Dystrophy (DMD) can present various challenges that impact the emotional well-being of individuals with the condition and their families. Coping strategies and support systems are crucial for navigating these challenges and maintaining a positive outlook. The following are key considerations for coping strategies and promoting emotional well-being in DMD:

Establishing a Supportive Network: Building a support network of family, friends, healthcare professionals, and support groups can provide emotional support, understanding, and practical assistance. Connecting with others who have similar experiences can be particularly valuable, as they can offer empathy, advice, and a sense of community.

Seeking Counseling or Therapy: Professional counseling or therapy can be beneficial for individuals with DMD and their families. Psychologists, social workers, or therapists with experience in chronic illness and disability can provide a safe space to discuss concerns, explore coping strategies, manage stress, and address emotional well-being. Therapy can help individuals develop resilience, enhance communication skills, and navigate the emotional challenges associated with DMD.

Developing Coping Skills: Identifying and practicing coping skills can help individuals manage stress and emotional challenges. This may include relaxation techniques, mindfulness exercises, deep breathing exercises, journaling, creative outlets (such as art or music), or engaging in hobbies or activities that bring joy and fulfillment. These strategies can help reduce anxiety, improve emotional well-being, and enhance overall resilience.

Open Communication: Open and honest communication within the family unit is crucial for maintaining emotional well-being. Encouraging open dialogue about feelings, concerns, and needs allows family members to support each other and address challenges collectively. Sharing information about DMD with extended family, friends, and school personnel can foster understanding and create a supportive environment.

Setting Realistic Goals: Setting realistic and achievable goals helps individuals with DMD maintain a sense of purpose and accomplishment.

Breaking larger goals into smaller, manageable steps can provide a sense of progress and prevent feelings of overwhelm. Celebrating successes, no matter how small, can contribute to a positive mindset and overall well-being.

Participating in Supportive Activities: Engaging in activities that promote well-being, such as physical exercise (within individual capabilities), hobbies, creative pursuits, or engaging with nature, can enhance mood, reduce stress, and provide a sense of fulfillment. Supportive activities that involve the whole family can strengthen bonds and create positive experiences.

Self-Care: Prioritizing self-care is essential for individuals with DMD and their caregivers. Taking time for relaxation, adequate rest, pursuing personal interests, and maintaining a healthy lifestyle can help manage stress, prevent burnout, and promote overall well-being. Caregivers should also seek support and respite care to ensure their own well-being.

Emotional Support for Siblings: Siblings of individuals with DMD may experience unique emotional challenges. Providing emotional support, open communication, and opportunities for siblings to express their feelings can help foster a healthy sibling relationship and reduce feelings of isolation or guilt.

7.2 Educational Support and Special Needs

Individuals with Duchenne Muscular Dystrophy (DMD) may require additional educational support and accommodations to ensure academic success and social inclusion. Collaborative efforts between families, educators, and healthcare professionals are crucial in meeting the educational needs of individuals with DMD. The following are key considerations for educational support and special needs:

Individualized Education Plan (IEP): Developing an Individualized Education Plan (IEP) is essential to address the specific learning needs and accommodations for individuals with DMD. The IEP outlines academic goals, specialized instruction, support services, and necessary accommodations, such as extended time for assignments or exams, physical accessibility, assistive technology, and modified physical education programs.

Accessibility and Physical Accommodations: Ensuring physical accessibility within the school environment is vital for individuals with DMD. This may involve wheelchair accessibility, ramps, elevators, accessible restrooms, and designated parking spaces. Adapting the classroom layout, furniture, and equipment to accommodate mobility aids and optimize participation is important.

Assistive Technology: Assistive technology plays a significant role in supporting individuals with DMD in their educational pursuits. It includes tools such as speech recognition software, text-to-speech programs, screen readers, adaptive keyboards, or alternative pointing devices. Evaluating the specific needs of the individual and providing appropriate assistive technology can enhance accessibility, communication, and learning opportunities.

Physical and Occupational Therapy in the School Setting: Collaborating with physical and occupational therapists can ensure the integration of therapy goals into the school environment. Therapy sessions may take place within the school setting, targeting specific functional goals, motor skills, mobility, and accessibility needs. Therapists can also provide guidance to school staff on safe transfers, positioning, and equipment use.

Peer Education and Sensitivity: Promoting peer education and sensitivity within the school community fosters understanding and inclusion. Educating classmates about DMD, its effects, and the abilities of individuals with DMD can reduce stigma, encourage empathy, and facilitate positive social interactions.

Transition Planning: Transition planning prepares individuals with DMD for the transition from school to adulthood. It involves discussing post-secondary education, vocational training, employment options, independent living skills, and accessing community resources. Collaboration between educators, healthcare professionals, and vocational counselors is crucial to ensure a smooth transition process.

Collaboration and Communication: Open communication and collaboration between families, educators, and healthcare professionals are vital for addressing the unique educational needs of individuals with DMD. Regular meetings, updates, and sharing relevant information ensure a cohesive approach to support academic success, monitor progress, and address any emerging challenges.

Social and Emotional Support: Providing social and emotional support within the school environment is important for the overall well-being of individuals with DMD. Encouraging inclusive activities, fostering peer relationships, and promoting a positive school culture that values diversity and empathy can enhance social integration and self-esteem.

It is essential to consider the individual needs, abilities, and preferences of each person with DMD when implementing educational support and accommodations. Regular evaluations, ongoing communication, and flexibility in approaches are key to ensuring a supportive and inclusive educational environment that promotes academic growth and social development.

Transitioning to adulthood and independence is an important milestone for individuals with Duchenne Muscular Dystrophy (DMD). Planning and support during this period are crucial to ensure a smooth transition and empower individuals to lead fulfilling lives. The following are key considerations for transitioning to adulthood and independence:

Transition Planning: Transition planning should begin early to allow sufficient time for preparation. It involves identifying goals, exploring post-secondary education options, vocational training, career planning, and independent living skills development. Collaboration between families, educators, healthcare professionals, and vocational counselors is essential to develop an individualized transition plan.

Vocational Counseling and Employment Support: Vocational counseling and employment support services can help individuals with DMD explore career options, identify strengths and interests, and develop skills necessary for employment. These services may include job coaching, resume building, interview preparation, and connecting individuals with job placement programs or supported employment opportunities.

Independent Living Skills: Developing independent living skills is crucial for individuals with DMD to achieve autonomy and self-sufficiency. This may involve learning skills such as managing personal care, financial management, meal planning and preparation, transportation, and accessing community resources. Occupational therapists and transition specialists can provide guidance and training in these areas.

Assistive Technology and Home Modifications: Utilizing assistive technology and making necessary home modifications can enhance independence and accessibility. This may include adaptive equipment, smart home technology, wheelchair ramps, grab bars, and accessible bathroom and kitchen features. Occupational therapists and assistive technology specialists can assess needs and recommend appropriate solutions.

Healthcare Transition: A smooth transition of healthcare from pediatric to adult providers is crucial. This involves identifying adult healthcare professionals experienced in managing DMD, ensuring continuity of care, and transferring medical records. It is important to address any specific healthcare needs, such as cardiac and respiratory monitoring, medication management, and coordination of multidisciplinary care.

Social Support and Peer Networks: Encouraging social support and fostering peer networks can contribute to a sense of belonging and community for individuals with DMD. Support groups, advocacy organizations, and social networks specifically for young adults with DMD provide opportunities for shared experiences, peer support, and mentorship.

Self-Advocacy and Decision-Making Skills: Building self-advocacy skills empowers individuals with DMD to express their needs, make informed decisions, and actively participate in their own care and life choices. Providing opportunities for decision-making, teaching self-advocacy strategies, and fostering independence gradually from a young age can help develop these skills.

Financial Planning and Benefits: Planning for financial security is important. Exploring financial assistance programs, disability benefits, and understanding financial management strategies can ensure individuals with DMD have the necessary resources to support their independence and quality of life. Financial advisors and support organizations can provide guidance in this area.

Transitioning to adulthood and independence requires careful planning, collaboration, and support from various stakeholders. Recognizing the unique strengths and abilities of individuals with DMD, promoting self-determination, and providing tailored resources and support services contribute to successful transitions and the achievement of perso

Advocacy and support organizations play a crucial role in the lives of individuals with Duchenne Muscular Dystrophy (DMD) and their families. These organizations provide a wealth of information, support, resources, and advocacy efforts to improve the quality of life for those affected by DMD. The following are key considerations regarding advocacy and support organizations:

Information and Resources: Advocacy organizations provide accurate and up-to-date information about DMD, treatment options, research updates, clinical trials, and available resources. They may publish educational materials, newsletters, and maintain comprehensive websites that serve as valuable sources of information for individuals with DMD and their families.

Support Networks and Peer Connections: Advocacy organizations often facilitate support networks and peer connections for individuals with DMD and their families. This can include support groups, online forums, social media communities, and events that bring together individuals facing similar challenges. These networks provide emotional support, share experiences, and offer a sense of community.

Parent and Family Support: Advocacy organizations recognize the needs of parents and families caring for individuals with DMD. They may offer specific support programs, counseling services, and resources to assist families in coping with the emotional, financial, and practical aspects of managing DMD. Parent-to-parent mentoring programs can also provide valuable guidance and support.

Educational Support and Advocacy: Advocacy organizations often play a crucial role in advocating for educational support and accommodations for individuals with DMD. They may provide guidance on navigating the educational system, developing Individualized Education Plans (IEPs), and ensuring that individuals with DMD receive appropriate educational services and accommodations.

Research Funding and Collaboration: Many advocacy organizations actively fund and promote research efforts to advance the understanding and treatment of DMD. They collaborate with researchers, healthcare professionals, and industry partners to support clinical trials, research studies, and the development of innovative therapies. Advocacy organizations also play a vital role in raising awareness about DMD among policymakers, healthcare providers, and the general public.

Legislative Advocacy: Advocacy organizations advocate for policy changes and legislation that benefit individuals with DMD and their families. They work to improve access to healthcare, insurance coverage, disability rights, inclusion in educational settings, and other areas that impact the lives of those affected by DMD. This advocacy helps shape public policy and ensures the voices of the DMD community are heard.

Collaboration with Healthcare Professionals: Advocacy organizations collaborate with healthcare professionals to promote best practices, disseminate information, and improve the coordination of care for individuals with DMD. These collaborations help ensure that individuals receive optimal medical care, have access to emerging therapies, and benefit from a multidisciplinary approach to care.

Awareness and Public Outreach: Advocacy organizations raise awareness about DMD and the challenges faced by individuals with the condition and their families. They organize awareness campaigns, events, and educational programs to promote understanding, inclusion, and support for the DMD community. These efforts help reduce stigma, increase public knowledge, and foster a supportive environment.

7.5 Future Outlook and Hope

The future outlook for individuals with Duchenne Muscular Dystrophy (DMD) is filled with hope due to ongoing research, advancements in medical treatments, and the tireless efforts of researchers, healthcare professionals, advocacy organizations, and the DMD community. The following are key considerations regarding the future outlook for DMD:

Innovative Therapies: Promising therapeutic approaches, such as gene therapies, exon skipping, gene editing, and regenerative medicine, are being developed and evaluated in clinical trials. These therapies have the potential to target the underlying cause of DMD, slow disease progression, and improve muscle function. Continued research and development may lead to more effective treatments and improved outcomes.

Early Intervention and Screening: Early diagnosis and intervention play a crucial role in managing DMD. Advances in newborn screening methods and improved understanding of the genetic basis of the condition enable early identification of affected individuals. Early intervention programs, such as physical therapy, corticosteroid treatment, and respiratory support, can help optimize outcomes and delay disease progression.

Multidisciplinary Care: The multidisciplinary care approach for DMD continues to evolve, focusing on comprehensive management and addressing the various aspects of the condition. Collaboration among healthcare professionals, including neurologists, cardiologists, pulmonologists, physical therapists, and occupational therapists, ensures a holistic approach to care and optimal management of DMD.

Clinical Trials and Research: Clinical trials play a crucial role in evaluating the safety and efficacy of emerging therapies for DMD. Ongoing research efforts focus on understanding the disease mechanisms, identifying new therapeutic targets, improving delivery methods, and developing innovative treatments. Continued participation in clinical trials contributes to the advancement of

DMD research and the development of more effective therapies.

Patient Advocacy and Empowerment: Advocacy organizations and the DMD community play a pivotal role in raising awareness, influencing policy changes, and promoting the needs and rights of individuals with DMD. Patient advocacy efforts help shape research priorities, improve access to care, and foster a supportive and inclusive environment for individuals with DMD and their families.

Quality of Life Enhancements: Efforts are being made to enhance the quality of life for individuals with DMD through the development of assistive technologies, improvements in accessibility, and the provision of psychosocial support services. These advancements aim to optimize independence, social inclusion, and overall well-being for individuals with DMD.

While challenges remain, the collective efforts of researchers, healthcare professionals, advocacy organizations, and the DMD community provide hope for the future. With continued progress, innovation, and collaboration, there is optimism for improved treatments, enhanced quality of life, and ultimately a cure for Duchenne Muscular Dystrophy.

Frequently Asked Questions (FAQs)

8.1 What is the life expectancy for individuals with Duchenne muscular dystrophy?

The life expectancy for individuals with Duchenne muscular dystrophy (DMD) has significantly improved over the years due to advancements in medical care and supportive therapies. In the past, individuals with DMD often did not survive beyond their teenage years or early 20s. However, with better management and interventions, many individuals with DMD are now living into their 30s, 40s, and beyond.

It's important to note that life expectancy can vary depending on several factors, including the individual's overall health, access to comprehensive care, the presence of complications such as cardiac or respiratory issues, and the specific genetic mutation causing DMD. Regular medical follow-ups, multidisciplinary care, proactive management of cardiac and respiratory function, and ongoing research advancements all contribute to improving life expectancy in individuals with DMD.

8.2 Can Duchenne muscular dystrophy be cured?

Currently, there is no known cure for Duchenne muscular dystrophy (DMD). However, research and clinical trials are focused on developing innovative treatments and therapies to address the underlying genetic cause of DMD and improve muscle function.

Emerging treatment approaches, such as gene therapies, exon skipping, gene editing, and regenerative medicine, hold promise for the future. These therapies aim to slow disease progression, restore or enhance dystrophin production, and improve overall muscle function. While these treatments are still in various stages of development and require further research, they offer hope for potential future cures for DMD.

In the meantime, the management of DMD focuses on multidisciplinary care, supportive therapies, and interventions to optimize quality of life, maintain function, and manage symptoms and complications associated with the condition.

8.3 Are there any dietary recommendations for DMD patients?

Maintaining a healthy and balanced diet is important for individuals with Duchenne muscular dystrophy (DMD). While there are no specific dietary recommendations exclusively for DMD, certain considerations can be helpful:

Adequate Caloric Intake: Individuals with DMD may have higher caloric needs due to increased energy expenditure and muscle wasting. Ensuring adequate caloric intake can help support overall nutrition and energy levels.

Balanced Diet: A balanced diet that includes a variety of foods from different food groups is important. This includes fruits, vegetables, whole grains, lean proteins, and healthy fats. Nutrient-dense foods can provide essential vitamins, minerals, and antioxidants.

Calcium and Vitamin D: Adequate calcium and vitamin D intake is important for maintaining bone health. Dairy products, fortified plant-based milk, leafy green vegetables, and supplements (under medical supervision) can help meet the calcium and vitamin D needs.

Protein: Protein is essential for muscle maintenance and repair. Including lean sources of protein such as poultry, fish, beans, lentils, tofu, and dairy products can help support muscle health.

Hydration: Maintaining adequate hydration is important for overall health. Encouraging regular fluid intake, preferably from water, helps prevent dehydration and supports proper bodily functions.

It is recommended to consult with a healthcare professional or a registered dietitian who specializes in neuromuscular disorders for personalized dietary guidance based on individual needs, preferences, and any specific considerations or restrictions.

8.4 How does Duchenne muscular dystrophy affect mental health?

Duchenne muscular dystrophy (DMD) can have an impact on mental health and well-being, both for individuals with DMD and their families. Some potential factors that can contribute to mental health challenges include:

Emotional Impact: Receiving a diagnosis of DMD and witnessing the progression of the condition can cause emotional distress, anxiety, grief, and sadness for individuals and their families.

Physical Limitations: The progressive loss of muscle strength and mobility can lead to frustration, loss of independence, and feelings of isolation or depression.

Social Challenges: Individuals with DMD may face social challenges, such as limited participation in certain activities, accessibility issues, and potential discrimination or stigma related to their condition. These factors can affect self-esteem and social interactions.

Caregiver Stress: Family members and caregivers of individuals with DMD often experience high levels of stress, balancing care giving responsibilities with other aspects of life. This can impact their own mental well-being.

It is essential to address mental health needs and promote emotional well-being in individuals with DMD and their families. Psychosocial support, counseling, support groups, and access to mental health services can be beneficial in managing emotional challenges and promoting overall mental well-being. Collaborating with healthcare professionals, support organizations, and mental health providers can help address these needs effectively.

www.ingramcontent.com/pod-product-compliance
Lightning Source LLC
Chambersburg PA
CBHW070851260726

48661CB00004B/1352